Hope
for
Health

Hope for Health

ILLUMINATING THE FOUNDATIONS OF HEALTH AND WELLNESS

JANET MADRID, BS, RDH

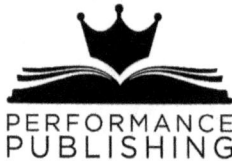

PERFORMANCE
PUBLISHING

Contents

Dedication

I dedicate this book first to God, for calling me into dentistry at age sixteen. I am so blessed to be in a profession whose mission is to improve the public's overall health and promote the dental hygiene profession as a highly valued and integral part of the healthcare system. I have been in this field for forty-five years and I am more passionate than ever about my part in promoting health and preventing disease.

To my family: my mother, who gave me a good work ethic and grit; my four wonderful daughters, Jessica, Sophia, Katherine, and Leolani, who studied with me during hygiene school and sat through lectures and slide presentations about all things dental hygiene and who make me more proud every day; my grandchildren, who eagerly listen to all my advice to them on teeth and health, you are my legacy; and to my husband, who is my biggest cheerleader, love of my life, and biggest supporter of my dream of having my own holistic dental hygiene practice. Thank you for making it possible for me to spread my message of *Hope for Health*.

To my fellow hygienists (my tribe) who mentor me, support me, and fight for their patients' lives every day. I can't begin to name you all. *You know who you are!*

To Dewitt Wilkerson DMD, author of *The Shift* and founder of the Integrative Dental Medicine Scholar Society (IDMSS), thank you for reigniting my passion for dental hygiene, and teaching me the importance of my role in dentistry as an oral-systemic disease prevention specialist. Your pursuit of integrating dentistry and medicine is truly inspirational.

To all the health practitioners, educators, and advocates who have been instrumental in my hundreds of hours of continuing education on all of the topics in this book, I salute your body of work. Without your research, inspiration, passion for education, and dedication to improving the health of the world, I would not be able to help my patients improve their health and quality of life.

And lastly, to Bernard Baros, DDS, who introduced me to a profession that I love and have dedicated my life to. I wish you could see how far I've come. Rest in peace.

Foreword

So many health books out there, right? That's not a bad thing, of course. But finding one that not only delivers the information you're looking for but also inspires real, actionable change? That's rare. This book is one of those rare finds—it struck me immediately after my first read.

The author is someone I deeply admire. And here's the twist: it's not a dentist. It's a dental hygienist. In Colorado, dental hygienists can practice independently—a unique and forward-thinking model I've always supported, even though parts of the profession see it as threatening. Personally, I think it's a win for everyone. It makes care more accessible, more affordable, and, as I learned at a recent meeting with dental hygienists from the Colorado Dental Hygienists Association (CODHA), it's about more than just cost. Often, it's literally about accessibility—bringing care to people who might otherwise not have the ability to get to a dental office due to transportation challenges. That fact was eye-opening for me.

And then there's the author, Janet. She's not just your typical dental hygienist. She's part of a small, exceptional group that not only educates patients in the dental office but also ties the oral-systemic connection into everything she does. She bridges the gap between oral health and systemic health in a way that's functional, forward-looking, and incredibly impactful. What makes her stand out even more is her ability to present this information in a way that's hopeful, digestible, and motivating.

Instead of overwhelming readers with endless details or to-do lists that make change feel impossible, Janet's approach feels attainable. It's positive. It's actionable. It's the kind of message that inspires movement instead of paralysis. For someone starting a health journey or looking to make meaningful lifestyle changes, this book is an incredible resource. It's not just a guide—it's something you'll come back to again and again for motivation and clarity.

This book integrates dentistry with holistic health, emphasizing the interconnectedness of oral and overall well-being. The author, with extensive clinical experience, advocates for preventative care and a functional, integrative approach to healthcare. She stresses the importance of foundational health practices—proper breathing, hydration, nutrition, movement, mindfulness, and strong social connections—to prevent and reverse chronic diseases. The text also highlights the crucial role of the oral microbiome in overall health and provides practical advice and resources for improving various aspects of well-being. Ultimately, the book aims to empower readers to take control of their health and live longer, healthier lives.

But here's what I find most encouraging: the irony—though it's not lost on me or other forward-thinking dentists and dental hygienists—is that this knowledge and clinical intelligence come from a dental hygienist. What better front-line healthcare professional to remind us that so many chronic diseases begin in the mouth? This book is a starting point, a spark to set you on a path toward better health, a longer lifespan, and a greater health span.

As a proud member of a professional dental organization that fosters clinicians and authors like Janet, I'm inspired by her vision and her ability to empower others through education and action. For anyone passionate about their health or the health of their patients, this book is an absolute must-read.

Mark Burhenne DDS,
Functional Dentist, Founder of *AskTheDentist* and *FYGG*

Foundation

"Life shrinks or expands in proportion to one's courage!"
Anais Nin

Sometimes you just need a manual. Every piece of equipment, automobile, technology, and gadget comes with an operator or owner's manual. I think every parent wishes they had one on how to raise another human. I know I did. But for whatever reason, God didn't see fit to give us one. We learn by the example of our parents and grandparents for better or worse.

As a young mother, I didn't have the internet or time to go to the library to search for answers. Thankfully, my girls survived my apprenticeship as a mother, and I learned a lot along the way. I worked with what I knew and hoped it was enough. There is a quote from Maya Angelou that says, *"Do the best you can until you know better. Then, when you know better, do better."* This message has given me comfort and grace for all the things I didn't do right in my own life and while raising my girls, and it is applicable to every area of my life.

The beautiful thing about life is that there is always hope for change. We always have a choice to learn from our mistakes and do better. We are a resilient and adaptable species. As long as we are still breathing, there is hope.

This book is about the big picture. The idea is that with an open mind and the desire to change the behaviors that harm our ability to adapt, there is *Hope for Health.*

As an oral systemic health professional, my overarching mission is to educate, equip, and empower my patients to improve their oral health and ultimately their overall health, because the mouth is connected to the rest of the body. This is an extensively researched and proven fact.

I am a lifelong learner and believe that education and learning never end. Research and technology continue to advance at warp speed. Thousands of researchers work diligently to understand all aspects of human anatomy and physiology, including its intricate metabolic processes and pathways down to the subatomic level. The sheer number of research papers published every day is mind-boggling.

Like many people today, I was skeptical about artificial intelligence (AI), worried that robots and computers would take over the world. Now, I realize the need for AI when it comes to interpreting and calculating data. AI is making it possible to leverage massive amounts of data to understand the complexities of human biology, thereby making it possible to understand the multifactorial causes of chronic disease and the potential for reversing it.

I have taken hundreds of hours of continuing education over the years, and I continue to try to keep up with the latest research and technology to serve my patients. Over the years there have been many shifts in how we previously thought about disease, its cause, and treatments. What we know now is that things are not as they once seemed. Remember when we were told not to eat eggs because of the cholesterol in them? That misinformation has been debunked. How about the "low fat" craze? We know now that we need good fat to build cells, especially the cells of our brains. We also need fat to utilize fat soluble vitamins like vitamins A, D, E, and K. I remember eating my salad with no dressing to avoid the fat. Little did I know that all those vitamins were not being absorbed because of the lack of fat dressing those beautiful veggies. How about when steaming broccoli or other vegetables was thought to be 'healthier'? I say add some real grass-fed butter to that broccoli and drizzle cold-pressed olive oil on that salad.

Today, we must keep an open mind and be willing to change our perspective about what we previously believed to be true in the ever-changing world of science and medicine. Yes, dentistry is oral medicine, and the last time I checked, the mouth is a part of the body. The mouth/body connection has been regrettably overlooked for too long. But change is on the horizon.

When I started my journey in dentistry, I didn't question the fact that medicine and dentistry were separate and even had separate insurance coverages. Like many things, I accepted it as a normal and logical fact. However, as my education, experience, and knowledge grew, I questioned the logic. After all, the mouth is part of the body, and an infection in the mouth or teeth affects the rest of the body, does it not? So, it is rational to say that any problem in the mouth is a medical problem.

Countless people have died from oral infections. My great-grandfather was one of them. In fact, many diseases are communicable and transmitted through saliva—diseases that, in fact, affect the whole body. Every oral disease affects the rest of the body and is medically necessary to treat. Therefore, they should be covered by medical insurance. Treatment of disease and health are basic human rights. I think we can all agree on this. However, some time ago medical and dental schools were separated, as were insurance plans to address medical and dental problems. I believe this was a big mistake, one that should be rectified. However, this subject has been debated for decades and is not the subject of this book. Just food for thought.

I am writing this book as a resource for my patients, friends, family, and anyone who wants to know better so they can do better for themselves, and those they love and care for. Have you heard the saying, "*If you do what you've always done, you'll get what you've always got?*" That is the truth, but we need to accept that we have all made mistakes and poor choices along life's path, but if we let go of the guilt and the blame of what was, we can have hope and faith in what can and will be.

As I previously stated, I am an oral health professional, and my mission and focus are disease prevention and health promotion. Contrary to what most people think, I am not a "tooth cleaner" (exclusively). Like I said before, research has proven that oral health is directly related to overall health. My role and the role of every dental professional is to educate, equip, and empower our patients to prevent, improve, and reverse oral disease, and, as a result, optimize their overall health, as members of their healthcare team.

This mission is not an easy one. It requires much education. In fact, the dental hygiene accrediting body requires 2,932 hours of education before a dental hygiene student can apply for licensure. Additionally, we must pass national, regional, and state boards, both written and practical. Believe it or not, all of these hours of education and rigorous testing aren't the hardest part. The hardest part is the critical thinking skills necessary to connect the dots for each patient based on their unique medical history, clinical presentation, immune health, diet, habits, behaviors, and testing. We must also be good listeners, detectives, researchers, clinicians, and occasionally hand holders. Every human is different—this is bio-individuality. It's not an easy profession to excel in. It's not for the faint of heart, the queasy, the apathetic, or the "I've learned all there is to know."

In dental hygiene school, we learned that an individual's immune response to a pathogen (the "host response") greatly affects whether disease will occur and to what extent. Did you know that at any given time, our bodies have cancer cells that are destroyed by our immune system before they can turn into full blown cancer? Our immune system is constantly seeking and destroying anything that is potentially harmful to us. As long as we support this system and don't interfere with its ability to protect and heal us, it will defend us!

However, the bio-individuality of each person is not the only confounding issue. The cause of each chronic disease is multifactorial, and environmental factors differ for each individual. It is pretty complicated. Genetics, the strength of one's immune system, and environmental stressors dictate whether an individual gets a disease and to what extent. The bad news is there is no one-size-fits-all, magic elixir, or silver bullet. Many factors need to be considered, and many dots have to be connected. You've heard the saying, *"It takes a village to raise a child,"* well, it takes a team to support the health of a human. No single provider has all the answers, nor can anyone be an expert in every area!

We all know the current model of disease management is not working to turn the tide of chronic disease. *But there is hope!* There is a new model of healthcare. A model that looks at the patient from a holistic perspective. One that looks for the root cause of disease, rather than just a treatment for symptoms. It is time to connect the mouth back to the rest of the body in order to integrate prevention and treatment through collaboration with all disciplines.

The American Academy of Oral Systemic Health (AAOSH), founded by Chris Kammer, DDS, says, "Collaboration cures." In healthcare, collaboration is when healthcare professionals with different backgrounds work together to provide the best outcome for the patient. Interdisciplinary organizations like AAOSH and the Integrative Dental Medicine Scholar Society (IDMSS), both of which I am a proud member, are leading the charge and championing the medical/dental integration movement with great success. The American Dental Association (ADA) has recently joined the cause to connect the mouth back to the body—*at last!* It is very important that all health practitioners know enough about how the body functions as a system to screen for potential problems that may require referral to another health practitioner that is more specialized in that area.

That is to say, medical doctors need to be able to screen for dental problems that may be linked to a medical problem they are finding and vice versa. Every health practitioner must consider the whole of the body. We must not treat the body myopically. We must consider the function of each system in relation to the whole. This is the essence of holistic, functional, and integrative approaches.

I am an "everything works out for the good," "the glass is half full," and "look for the silver lining" type of girl. Optimism is my middle name. *I am a hope generator!* My goal, and the purpose of this book is to give people hope that health is possible, and disease can be optional, depending on their choices.

The information I present is not medical advice and I don't claim to know everything or have all the answers. My hope is that the information I share with you will raise your awareness of what constitutes health and wellness and how it is connected to the mouth and to every behavior and choice we make everyday. I hope this information will pique your curiosity to do a deeper dive into the area that interests you or that you are being challenged in.

I will be providing you with many resources, which are not exhaustive by any means, but are keys to the answers you may be looking for. Thanks to the internet, there is more information available than I can hope to share or even explore in my lifetime. However, for the curious, adventurous, and ever hopeful, the journey that is possible through the exploration of the topics I present has endless possibilities.

CHAPTER 1

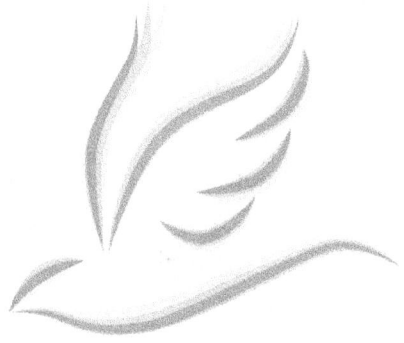

Genesis

"The doctor of the future will give no medicine,
but will interest his patient in the human frame,
in diet and in the cause and prevention of disease."
– Thomas Edison, 1903

Let's get started. I want this book to be an easy read and a quick reference manual of sorts. I am not going to bore you with a bunch of statistics and deep science. You will be able to find those things in the resources I cite later on. We are all too aware of the staggering rise in chronic disease and the exorbitant number of deaths that are related to cardiovascular disease, Alzheimer's disease, dementia, cancer, Parkinson's, and diabetes, to name a few. I won't debate where the blame lies. We know modernization, Big Pharma, Big Food, Big Ag, and Big Government have all contributed in their own way. Not to mention the pervasive greed and corruption associated therein.

Let's focus on where we are now and what can be done. I want to generate hope and illuminate ways to improve our health and healthspan. Lifespan does not account for quality of life. Someone can live a long time on medications or in a declining state of illness where they can't care for themself at the most basic level. They may be alive, but have no autonomy, memory, mobility, or the ability to communicate. Basically, they can be alive with no quality of life. I don't know anyone who would want to "live" like that. Our goal should be increasing our healthspan. Healthspan is the ability to live a long time in health with strength, mobility, cognitive ability, and autonomy.

We now have the science, research, technology, and artificial intelligence that can be used for good to change the prevalence of chronic disease. Out with the old, outdated, and erroneous information of the recent past and in with the idea of getting back to the basics, back to the way God intended us to live with abundant health and well-being.

Focusing on prevention and root causes can target interventions that can reverse disease. Yes, even Alzheimer's disease (ALD) is being reversed thanks in part to the work of people like Dale Bredesen, MD, the author of *The End of Alzheimer's Program* and Richard Isaacson, MD, author of *The Alzheimer's Prevention and Treatment Diet*. A myriad of research is being done to end the epidemic of chronic disease, mostly with new drugs, but many others are working to educate the public on prevention and ways to improve our health and lives. *There is hope!* The information is out there. But it needs to be distilled down, and the dots need to be connected to help the public understand that they have the power to live a longer healthier life.

Contrary to what my mother, her mother, and many people have espoused, we are not victims of our biology. Just because your parent or grandparent had diabetes, arthritis, or heart disease, does not sentence you to the same plight. This is because of what we know from the science related to genetics and epigenetics.

Epigenetics is the ability to make changes in our environment, diet, and behaviors that will dictate whether genes are turned on or off. Genes do not change, but their expression is dependent on many factors that we can control and some that we can't (like the one billion pounds of pesticides sprayed on our crops per year—but people are working on that). DNA represents the genetic material of what is possible in the body, but from a functional standpoint, the presence of a gene doesn't mean it is active or *turned on*. In fact, mRNA represents what is actually happening in the body; it tells us what genes are actively being expressed.

AI is being leveraged by companies like Viome Health Science, that analyzes mRNA data from saliva, blood, and stool samples, so that they can offer highly-individualized health and wellness information to prevent and manage chronic disease. This type of cutting-edge technology is available to the public and is one of many technologies that give me hope for improved health on a global scale. Naveen Jain, one of the founders of Viome, believes that with this type of technology, "Disease is optional." In other words, there is always hope.

Our bodies are a miraculous superorganism with many biomes of microorganisms that live in and on us. The health and diversity of these microbiomes are critical for the health of the human body. Kiran Krishnan, renowned clinical research microbiologist says, "People have so much more control over their health and wellness than they think. Most diseases are derived from a dysfunctional ecosystem. We can fix the ecosystem and that will give us a much better position on our wellness." Leveraging these microbiomes is entirely possible now thanks to an abundance of research on this topic and companies like Microbiome Labs, which produce quality spore-based probiotics that can help recondition and restore the gut to health.

We are an adaptable species that has an innate ability to heal when given the proper support. Living in health is a basic right and achieving health shouldn't require costly drugs or procedures. For example, a drug was developed to treat people with Alzheimer's disease. The cost of that drug was $56,000 per year for the patient, and it was found to be ineffective. There have been over four hundred of these drugs developed for ALD, all of which have been ineffective and lay in a massive graveyard of failed drugs. I firmly believe the amount of money being spent on drugs to address symptoms of disease could be spent on prevention and have a bigger impact.

Believe it or not, health can be virtually free. Redirecting our resources, time, and energy from things that harm our health to things that promote our health can change the trajectory of our lives. It is easier than you think. For instance, breathing (air is still free, for now), taking a walk barefoot, exercising, swimming, meditating, singing, humming, dancing, sitting in the sun, volunteering, sleeping, and spending time with the people you love or care about, just to name a few.

None of these things have to cost anything and there isn't any money to be made with these free activities (unless you have no imagination and want to pay for them, i.e., gym memberships, eating out, etc.). Therein lies the problem, whether it is marketable or profitable, stakeholders of public health, the government, etc., are not focusing on these free and effective promoters of health on a large scale.

Someone told me recently that, "Without money there is no mission." This is sad and I don't agree. However, the mission of obliterating chronic disease will save a lot of money for the people paying for multiple prescription drugs. Only the entities making money from people who are chronically ill will be losing.

Trillions of dollars are being spent on finding drugs that are purported to be the silver bullets for the chronic diseases that are epidemic worldwide. These endeavors are futile because monotherapies (single treatments) for chronic disease don't work when these chronic diseases have many different factors that contribute to it and vary from person to person. People are bio-individual. They have different genetics, different environments, different behaviors, and different physiology. The fix is not quick. It requires patience, persistence, and flexibility.

As I said before, people need a team to help them prevent disease or help them regain their health once it is lost, and that team needs a quarterback. They need a health practitioner that screens for disease as early as possible, helps them navigate the tests required, and refers them to other health practitioners when appropriate. In many cases, these quarterbacks can be found in the field of dentistry. According to Mike Czubiak, DDS, author of *Hygiene Superstar*, dental hygienists who are highly skilled and knowledgeable health advocates can contribute not only to the oral health of their patients but also to the broader systemic health issues that can be screened for and identified in a dental hygiene visit. We have the opportunity to support our patients with early health strategies to improve their overall health outcomes.

This is "whole health" dentistry. Dentistry from a holistic perspective. It is a functional and integrative approach, which is precision and individualized medicine that collaborates with other health practitioners for the good of the patient. Complete health is possible with the right mindset, motivation, and team members. I can't overstate the importance of the choices we make now in how healthy our future will be. Medical Dental Integration is key.

My mom used to say, *"Don't let yourself go because it's hard to get it back when you're old."* Peter Attia, MD, author of *Outlive: The Science & Art of Longevity*, says that we need to start saving now for our retirement years or, as he puts it, our "Centenarian Decathlon", which is our last decade of life. His book delves into the science of longevity and, as a physician, he discusses in depth things like heart rate variability (HRV), nutritional biochemistry, cardiovascular disease, cancer prevention, and exercise physiology, to name a few.

One of the most profound statements he makes in his book's *epilogue* is something I firmly believe. It is a quote from his friend, Ric Elias, a survivor of the US Airways flight that landed in the Hudson River in 2009. He said, "I think people get old when they stop thinking about the future." I find this so true. People who look at life as though their best years are behind them have no motivation to live out a better life going forward. If you are reading this book, you are not one of those people. The best is yet to come.

Think about it, our creator equipped our bodies and our environment with all that we need to live an abundantly long and healthy life. Our home, planet Earth, has everything we need to thrive, and he put us in charge of taking care of it and the life on it. *How are we doing with that?* Not very well, considering the state of the environment and the state of our collective health.

But don't lose hope, the components of health and longevity are not really a mystery. Our ancestors managed very well; unless they were killed by a predator, wounded in battle, or died from a subsequent infection or from complications of childbirth, life was easy.

They had clean air to breathe, and clean water to drink. They were able to grow, kill, or catch whatever they needed to eat. They went to sleep and woke up with the rising and setting of the sun. Their everyday life required physical activity. In a sense it was a simpler life.

However, there are many benefits to our modern life; being killed by a predator is not very likely (notwithstanding the possibility of being intentionally or accidentally killed by someone or something); dying from an infection is not likely due to the advent of antibiotics (despite the consequences of their overuse: superbugs); and although the morbidity and mortality rate in childbirth in the US is higher than other parts of the world (despite our higher dollars being spent), it is likely lower than our ancestors. But sadly, we have engineered ourselves into a lifestyle that has replaced most of what was the day-to-day, natural, healthy lifestyle of our ancestors.

The air we breathe is still free (for now), but it isn't clean. We have to pay for water that is no longer pure, an optimal pH, and is lacking essential minerals. Most of us don't grow, gather, hunt, or catch our own food. Movement has become virtually unnecessary. Many of us have to rely on technology to make sure we take enough steps in our day. We don't even have to cook, and food can be delivered "ready to eat" right to our door. Shopping and working can be done from home. *Convenience? Or a recipe for chronic disease?*

While our ancestors may have had shorter lifespans because of the high rate of sudden death, long lives were generally lived in a state of health. Chronic disease, as we know it today, didn't exist unless you were royalty and lived life in excess and had servants and doctors that could rudimentarily prolong your life of suffering.

Modern man's life span has increased because of medicine. Medical intervention and pharmacology have increased our lifespan, but not our health span. Health is not the mere absence of disease. The World Health Organization (WHO) defines health as *"a state of complete physical, mental, and social well-being."* They further define well-being as a state that encompasses a *"quality of life and the ability of people and societies to contribute to the world with a sense of meaning and purpose."* Having a purpose is a huge key to healthful longevity.

Have you ever thought about how many people would not be alive today in nursing homes, assisted living, and even in the care of loved ones, if it were not for polypharmacy? If given the choice, would you choose quantity of years lived or quality of life?

Why should you have to choose? The following chapters cover what I believe (and what my education and research has taught me) are the fundamental and foundational components of health and the simple and practical ways that you can explore and apply them to your life.

BODY

CHAPTER 2

Breathe

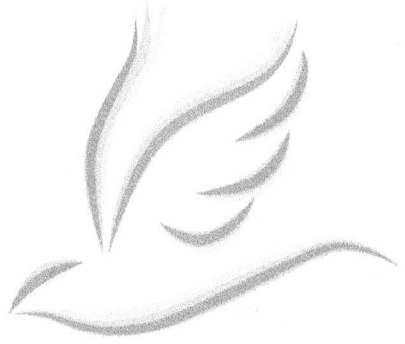

"The Lord God formed the man from the soil of the earth.
He breathed the breath of life into man's nostrils,
and the man became a living being."
Genesis 2:7

I moved from Hawaii back to Colorado with my four girls in tow to go to dental hygiene school in 1996. As a full-time student and single mom, my finances were less than optimal. We lived in some very cramped, dare I say, sketchy quarters (sorry, girls). However, the two-bedroom apartment for the five of us was a blessing in disguise. I started to notice that my youngest daughter Leolani, who was not quite two, was snoring and having difficulty breathing when she slept. I also noticed her chest was caving in as she gasped for air. It was quite frightening. I took her to the pediatrician who sent us to an Ear Nose and Throat doctor (ENT), who said they didn't see anything wrong with her except that she had another ear infection, which ultimately resulted in multiple rounds of antibiotics and sets of tubes.

She eventually had to have "permanent" tubes in her ears, which made her very sensitive to loud sounds.

However, even after the tubes were placed, the distressed breathing at night persisted. I thought there had to be something else. I didn't know anything about sleep apnea or how to screen for it at that time, so I took her for a second opinion to another ENT. The doctor said the caving in of her chest was called pectus excavatum as if it was normal. I asked him if her tonsils and adenoids were affecting her breathing and snoring. He said they were enlarged but he didn't recommend removing them because she hadn't had multiple bouts of strep throat.

She was still mouth breathing at night and I remembered the book *Atlas of the Mouth* that Dr. Baros gave me to study, back when I started working for him as a dental assistant in the late 1970s. There was a sketch of the profile of a mouth breather that had a small recessed chin, and forward head posture and I didn't want her to end up looking like that. I didn't realize at that time that the lack of oxygen to her brain was the more serious health concern. Looking back, she had more signs that I wasn't aware of. She had dark circles under her eyes, which is called venous pooling, a typical sign of sleep-disordered breathing in children and adults. She was often tired and grouchy, which I attributed to being a toddler and our hectic schedule.

The ENT and I went back and forth, until he finally agreed to take her tonsils out but not her adenoids. Her breathing at night improved somewhat but was still labored. She ended up having to have a second surgery to take her adenoids out. I was very upset that she had to be put under general anesthesia a second time because that ENT didn't know what I now know about the importance of airway in childhood development. Looking back, I believe there was an allergy component that caused her to mouth breathe, because I just learned she has allergies and her nose is frequently stuffy. We're working on that.

This story is not an unfamiliar one. Thankfully, what we know today is that enlarged tonsils and adenoids in children are a detriment to their health because they compromise their airway and are largely a result of mouth breathing. Tonsils get inflamed when they are trying to filter the air that is normally filtered through the nose. Allergies are often the culprit in mouth breathing. Thankfully, ENTs are more airway-focused now, for the most part. ENTs that refuse to remove tonsils and adenoids for compromised airways are hopefully the exception and not the rule.

It is not common knowledge, but children can have sleep-disordered breathing (SDB) and sleep apnea. It is not only a problem of the overweight, thick-necked, middle-aged man. Everyone, but especially children, should be screened as early as possible by knowledgeable dental and medical professionals, lactation consultants, pediatricians, and orofacial myologists. It is our duty and obligation as dental health professionals to screen for signs of compromised airways. We don't learn a lot about this in dental or dental hygiene school because the curriculum is often decades behind. However, there is ample opportunity for advanced education on this and other disease prevention topics. I, for one, am thankful for all the opportunities to get more education related to health and prevention of disease. Although I take multiple courses every month, I wish I had more time and resources to learn even more.

Oxygen is life. The human body is complex and consists of many elements and building blocks. The most abundant element in the human body is oxygen. It makes up approximately sixty-five percent of our bodies. Unlike other elements, it cannot be stored for a long time in the body. A constant supply is needed by all of our cells and tissues to live.

Without oxygen our body cannot build new cells to replace old ones or even function, for that matter. All cells have different lifespans; for example, skin cells can live for two to three weeks, while red blood cells live for about four months. Brain cells are thought to be able to live longer than a human, up to two hundred years, but not without oxygen. Imagine that! Our brain cells can live up to two hundred years, yet we aren't living up to our potential.

According to the National Institute of Health (NIH), the brain can be irreversibly damaged after three to four minutes without oxygen, and any longer than that, death is imminent. So, oxygen is arguably the most vital element for life. Ideally, our blood should be saturated with above 95% oxygen. Below 90% is considered too low. People with inadequate or compromised airways desaturate (decrease oxygen in the blood) to levels below 90% multiple times per night, compromising their health. When hospitalized, a person whose oxygen goes below 90% is a cause for alarms to go off and the patient to be put on oxygen. It is a serious problem.

Like most people, I never knew the number of functions of oxygen to the human body. Did you know that oxygen is the number one source of energy/fuel for our bodies? Only 10% of our energy comes from food and water, while 90% comes from oxygen! I find this incredible. Additionally, many of the whole foods we eat contain oxygen. One more reason to eat whole foods. It is amazing how key oxygen is to life. It also aids in detoxifying our blood, strengthening our immune system, and enhancing the absorption of nutrients (think water soluble).

One of the things that is particularly important to oral health practitioners is that oxygen destroys anaerobic bacteria, parasites, and viruses. Ozone (O3), which is three molecules of oxygen, is a very strong antimicrobial. When used correctly, it doesn't harm healthy cells. However, breathing straight ozone can harm lung cells, so therapeutic use must be done with caution. This is why it is used extensively in holistic and biological dentistry. Other benefits of the use of ozone in dentistry include upregulating the immune system, increasing circulation, and helping the body heal.

Oxygen is not only essential to our brain for learning, feeling, and acting; it also helps calm our central nervous system. Hypoxia (oxygen deficiency) increases our heart rate and respiration because the heart has to work harder to get the oxygen it needs. Prolonged or severe hypoxia leads to heart and lung failure. Maintaining optimal oxygen levels equals health, vitality, physical stamina, and endurance. Without oxygen we are dead. It is vital to life.

Correct breathing is crucial for getting the oxygen we need, but like many processes of our body, breathing is one that is taken for granted. Frankly, we don't have to think about breathing. It is automatic. *Have you ever thought about how you breathe? Do you breathe through your nose or through your mouth?* Humans are obligate nasal breathers. This means that nasal breathing is a physiological instinct.

Mouth breathing is an emergency backup system. We are not meant to breathe through our mouths. Mouth breathing does not allow for proper tongue posture, which is resting in the roof of our mouth, and sealing off the throat for proper nasal breathing. If the tongue lies on the floor of the mouth and the mouth hangs open to breath, this changes the entire facial structure and development of the upper and lower jaw along with the sinuses that are located in the upper jaw. The roof of the mouth is the floor of the sinuses. Nasal breathing is crucial to our overall health. Optimal breathing is achieved when lips are closed, and the tongue is suctioned to the roof of the mouth.

There are many functions of the nose in addition to smelling. It prepares the air we breathe to be used by our bodies. It regulates the volume of air we take in. It filters, warms, and humidifies the air before it reaches our lungs, and it makes nitric oxide. Nitric oxide (not nitrous oxide, aka laughing gas) is a signaling molecule and is needed for many functions in the body. It also is an antimicrobial in the nasal passages. Nitric oxide has two production pathways. One is through nasal breathing, and one is through the digestion of nitrate in our diet which is broken down by good bacteria on the back of our tongue.

Rinsing with a strong antimicrobial mouthwash can kill these bacteria, lowering the amount of nitric oxide we can produce, which ultimately leads to endothelial dysfunction. From a dental standpoint, the use of antimicrobial mouth rinses should be discontinued and tongue brushing or scraping should be done instead. Tongue brushing and tongue scraping enhances the growth of the nitrate-reducing bacteria (good guys) on the tongue. The reason this is significant is because nitric oxide in a vasodilator and therefore helps regulate our blood pressure among many other very important functions in the body. As a signaling molecule and neurotransmitter, it is critical for communication between cells.

Dr. Louis Ignarro won a Nobel prize for the discovery of nitric oxide and its importance in the body. Nitric oxide has been coined the 'miracle molecule.' Nathan Bryan, PhD, who worked closely with Dr. Ignarro, and educates on all the functions of nitric oxide in the body, wrote a great book called *Functional Nitric Oxide Nutrition*. His book illuminates the importance of nutrition in producing adequate nitric oxide.

Another important reason for nasal breathing is that our nasal passages are lined with mucus that traps dust, bacteria, viruses, fungi, and other pollutants. Then cilia, which are tiny hairs that also line the nasal passage, sweep the mucous to the back of the throat so that it can be swallowed and neutralized by stomach acid (if it is strong enough).

Many people that suffer from acid reflux take antacids that reduce stomach acid, which allows some of the pathogens to survive and pass to the small intestine. This is one of the many problems that lead to dysbiosis in the gut, a problem that will be discussed in Chapter 4.

So, if we are obligate nasal breathers, why do many people breathe through their mouths? I illuminated one of the reasons with the story of my daughter. But, just like most things relating to the human body, there are multiple reasons.

Studies of the evolution of the human skull over time have revealed that our jaws, both the upper and lower jaw, are not developing as big as they once were. Consequently, the nasal cavity and sinuses are also getting smaller, making it more difficult for people to breathe through their nose, and making it easier for allergens to get trapped in cramped nasal turbinates.

Weston A. Price, DDS, studied this phenomenon throughout the world in the 1930s. He found that the reason behind this was because of the *civilization of men*. His book *Nutrition and Physical Degeneration* highlights the adverse effects of sugar, as well as refined and highly processed foods, not only from a standpoint of nutrition, but from a standpoint of jaw and facial development. Dr. Price names a lack of breastfeeding that stimulates proper growth and development of the jaws and a lack of chewing hard foods as the reason jaws are not developing to the optimal size. Chewing hard food like carrots, celery, nuts and apples stimulates this growth. Pureed foods, cereals and other soft foods along with the use of pacifiers, sippy cups and straws during growth and development puts the forces of the lips and cheeks working against this growth and development. Muscle trumps bone.

With smaller jaws, comes narrow and high vaulted palates (roof of the mouth), resulting in smaller sinuses (the palate is the floor of the sinuses), and deviated septums. When the roof of the mouth is highly arched instead of wide, the nasal septum is pushed up and can be deviated from the optimal midline position. This craniofacial underdevelopment makes it difficult to breathe through the nose.

Often there are associated orofacial myofunctional disorders that need to be addressed, such as improper swallow patterns, poor tongue tone and posture. Orofacial Myofunctional Therapists (OMTs) are essentially physical therapists of the mouth and facial muscles who help individuals overcome these disorders and work with individuals with tethered oral tissues such as tongue-ties or lip-ties, pre- and post-release, to ensure proper tongue tone and posture. There are great educational airway organizations that are putting out advanced training courses in improving airways through various means. Airway Health Solutions, The Breathe Institute, and The Vivos Institute are some that I have learned from. There are many treatments available. Everything from expansion of palates to rescue appliances that can replace a CPAP machine for sleep apnea.

The presence of a tongue-tie interferes with proper speech, but not always. It can affect a baby's ability to properly latch in nursing and prevent proper tongue posture in swallowing and breathing. This can lead to problems like colic and spitting up. It can also lead to tension in the neck, shoulders, and upper chest resulting in postural problems. I never knew that the fascia that connects the tongue to the floor of the mouth is connected to all the fascia of the rest of the body down to the toes. If the tongue is "tied" it creates tension throughout the body.

Dental professionals are in a unique position to be able to screen for this. A tongue-tie can be released with a laser and should be preceded and followed by orofacial myofunctional therapy. Retraining the tongue to function properly is very important when dealing with tongue and lip-ties, otherwise known as tethered oral tissues. Just like you need physical therapy for a broken arm that has been in a sling or a leg that has been in a cast, a tongue that has had limited mobility because of being tied to the floor of the mouth, will need physical therapy to learn proper movement for proper swallowing and nasal breathing.

One of the saddest things related to sleep apnea in children is that symptoms of sleep apnea are similar to those of ADD and ADHD. Kids who do not receive adequate oxygen when they sleep have irritability, lack of focus, and fatigue and are often misdiagnosed and put on medications. Parents who are being told that their child is exhibiting ADD or ADHD behaviors should have them evaluated for sleep and airway issues first. A good book to read is "*Sleep Wrecked Kids*" by Sharon Moore. It helps parents learn what good sleep looks like in their kids and how to look for the red flags for sleep problems. There will be more information about this book in Chapter 9.

As I stated before, mouth breathing is a major contributor to underdeveloped upper or lower jaws, which leads to an underdeveloped airway. Breathing through the mouth decreases the amount of oxygen available to tissues to the tune of a forty percent reduction. An underdeveloped airway can lead to some form of sleep-disordered breathing (SDB), like sleep apnea. You may think that an underdeveloped jaw is irreversible. The good news is that the expansion of the jaws to increase the airway is possible.

Old school orthodontics was mainly a retractive process. Removing permanent teeth that there wasn't room for and moving the teeth inward to close the space made the jaw even smaller than before. This practice has spawned an avalanche of undiagnosed sleep apnea. There are roughly twenty-four million undiagnosed cases in the US alone. This is putting a substantial economic burden on the healthcare system and is contributing to lost productivity and accidents.

The more current philosophy of orthodontics is one of expansion, because of what we know are airway issues stemming from the previous retractive methods. Crowded teeth are a sign of underdeveloped arches, and the first thought should be expansion—not pulling teeth. It is ideal to catch underdevelopment as soon as possible, preferably before the age of four to more easily guide growth, but improvement can be made at virtually any age with the proper treatment. If signs of SDB are caught early, simple guided-growth appliances can be used to help enlarge a child's jaws and airway in a short period of time. Many dentists are getting advanced training to focus on airways to improve the overall health of their patients. Granted, there are not enough practicing this way, but thankfully, the importance of airway in dentistry is on the rise. With increased awareness of the public comes increased demand for more practitioners to receive advanced training.

In fact, the ADA put out a policy statement in 2017, that addressed the fact that dental professionals are in an ideal position to screen for signs of SDB. The signs that present themselves in the head, neck, and oral cavity include retruded chins, narrow jaws, a tongue that hides the throat when the mouth is open, enlarged tonsils, scalloping on the sides of the tongue, wear of teeth, notching of teeth at the gumline, clenching and grinding, jaw joint pain, crowded teeth, periodontal disease, cavities, dry mouth, and mouth breathing. Individuals with these issues need to have a sleep study done to find out if any type of SDB is present and to what extent.

Sleep studies are easier and more convenient than they used to be. They can be administered at home now at a very low cost. Airway-focused dentists can administer home sleep studies via rings or wrist devices that can be read by a sleep physician for a diagnosis. If you or someone you love has any of the above signs of possible SDB you should talk to your primary care physician about a sleep study or see an airway-focused dentist that can evaluate your airway.

Contrary to what most people believe, proper breathing is slow through the nose with a low volume. According to Patrick McKeown in his book *Close Your Mouth*, over-breathing, which is generally through the mouth with "big" breaths, is basically a state of hyperventilation. When we hyperventilate, we lower carbon dioxide levels in the blood. Carbon dioxide plays a crucial role in delivering oxygen to our organs and tissues, a phenomenon known as the Bohr Effect. Ironically, the more air we take in, the less oxygen actually reaches our organs and tissues. I know—it blew my mind too. Not only does slower nasal breathing increase the amount of oxygen to our body, but it also calms our nervous system. Chronic hyperventilation signals our body that we are in distress. This raises stress hormones like cortisol and can lead to weight gain and anxiety. Slow low volume nasal breathing can help reduce cortisol and anxiety.

Did you know that carbon dioxide is also made when you exercise and digest your food? It is a byproduct of cellular respiration with a purpose. It helps regulate the pH in our blood, it helps bind oxygen to hemoglobin for delivery, and it helps dilate our airway and blood vessels. The carbon dioxide we don't use gets exhaled. And as in the circle of life, plants need the carbon dioxide we exhale to grow. We need plants and plants need us. We need the oxygen they produce through photosynthesis (plants metabolic pathway), and they need the carbon dioxide we produce through cellular respiration (humans' metabolic pathway).

Of course, the air we breathe should ideally be clean. With an increase in global pollution both indoors and outdoors, we must be good stewards of our environment. I won't get into environmental pollution, because it is not something we can easily control as individuals, although our choices as individuals can make an impact if enough of us are making good choices. There are certainly things we can do to do our part for our outdoor environment, but I want to discuss an area we don't think about much, our indoor environment. We have a lot of control over our indoor environment, mainly in our home and maybe not as much in our workplace.

I learned this the hard way. When I was twenty, I had a major life-threatening health issue. The extensive toxins I was exposed to in the dental office in the late seventies and early eighties caused my liver to shut down. I didn't know the reason till thirty years later and thankfully I lived to tell about it, but this realization motivated me to get out of conventional dentistry and start a holistic dental hygiene practice where I could protect myself and my patients.

You see, personal protective equipment (PPE) was not used when I started dentistry. Gloves and masks were not required. We simply washed our hands. As a young girl, of sixteen, I was exposed to lots of chemicals and their vapors along with mercury and its vapors. I also had multiple mercury fillings put in my mouth during that time and actually handled mercury daily with my bare hands. We used to squeeze the amalgam (powdered metals + liquid mercury) into a cheese cloth to get the excess mercury out to make it a specific consistency. At that time, I didn't know mercury was toxic. I confess, in my ignorance, I used to play with it. I thought it was cool when it would bead up into tiny little shiny balls.

In 2020, I learned about the toxicity of mercury and a lot about holistic and biological dentistry. The lightbulb went off as to why my liver failed when I was twenty. Thankfully, I was young, and healthy and, because the liver is a resilient and regenerative organ and my family prayed a lot, I recovered and didn't need a new liver. It was actually pretty miraculous.

We are exposed to more toxins and pollution than we know. According to the NIH, household air pollution has a significant negative impact on health worldwide in both developed and developing nations, but for different reasons. It affects every age group from conception to death and affects multiple body systems.

There are nearly sixty sources of household air pollution. In developing countries poor indoor air quality is due mainly to fuel sources for cooking. However, in developed countries the sources vary from smoking, household cleaners, pesticides, air fresheners, candles, furniture, and construction materials that emit volatile organic compounds (VOC's). Compounds from these sources are considered endocrine disruptors and obesogens. Ironically, people with more financial resources suffer the most from these endocrine disrupters because they are able to repaint their walls, buy new carpet and new furniture more often and purchase all the fancy air fresheners and candles to make their home smell nice.

Endocrine disrupting chemicals can interfere with hormone production and function, causing numerous health problems including infertility in both men and women. Think of all the in vitro fertilization (IVF) that is needed today.

Obesogens are types of endocrine disrupting chemicals that contribute to metabolic syndrome and obesity. Overall, these household pollutants are toxic to us. We need to become more aware of things in our home that are adversely affecting our health. Efforts to detoxify our home environment can pay dividends in improved health.

If you don't know what environmental toxins in your home could be, the Environment Working Group (EWG) is a great resource for finding out which foods and products are considered safe or unsafe (toxic) to the environment and for human consumption. They have a list of toxic chemicals to avoid, which are:

- BPA's – found in plastics and resins that mimic estrogen.
- Dioxins – from industrial waste and pollution that ultimately end up in our food.
- Atrazine – found in herbicides that also end up in our food and water.
- Phthalates – found in plastics and some personal care products.
- Perchlorate – from rocket fuel that can be found in food and water.
- Fire retardants – found in furniture, carpet and padding, and some clothing.
- Lead – found in old paint, old pipes and water; arsenic-found in water.
- Mercury – found in silver fillings and some fish.
- PFC's – found in non-stick cookware, upholstery, tent material, and clothing.
- Organophosphates – found in pesticides and conventionally farmed produce.

It's pretty scary how much we are exposed to toxic chemicals. The EWG has an app that has the capability to look up hundreds of products to see if they are safe.

* * * * *

Meditation, breathing exercises, and breath work are becoming increasingly popular due in part to the works of James Nestor in his book *Breathe* and Patrick McKeown in his book *The Oxygen Advantage*. Adding an intentional practice of breathing exercises can improve your respiratory health, reduce stress and anxiety, improve cardiovascular health, help you lose weight, and promote better sleep.

Mouth taping is a practice that helps people retrain themselves to breathe through their nose. Many people breathe through their mouths out of habit. If you have severe allergies that cause chronic sinusitis and congestion, you may not be able to breathe through your nose, so mouth taping would be inappropriate until your allergies and chronic congestion are resolved.

Close Your Mouth, also by Patrick McKeown, has exercises for overcoming chronic sinusitis and asthma. A colleague that I admire and have learned a lot from in the area of nasal breathing and craniofacial development is Trish O'Hehir, MS, RDH. In her book *LipZip: Breathe Better to Live Better*, she discusses all things nasal breathing in an easy pocket handbook format. I often give a copy to my patients.

Additionally, there are new methods of treating allergies long-term that can be accessed virtually and do not involve pricking your back with allergens and weekly shots. Sublingual Immunotherapy (SLIT) can be administered by an allergist via telehealth upon submitting a self-administered "blood spot" fingerstick test that reveals what you are allergic to. Then, specific personalized drops are formulated and mailed to the patient which are administered under the tongue daily at home instead of weekly shots. One such company is Wyndly, which can be accessed directly online to the consumer.

There is a ton of information about the importance of proper breathing and the need for oxygen. Start paying attention to your breathing and of those around you. You'll be surprised how many people you will see that are mouth breathing.

A common phrase people use when trying to help someone who is stressed is 'just breathe.' It reminds me of a song I like by Jonny Diaz called Breathe, which talks about how chaotic life can be and the importance of slowing down to 'just breathe.' It's one of the best ways to calm your nervous system.

Key Points:

- **Remember, slow and calm breathing helps regulate our nervous system.**
- Breathe through your nose at all times (when awake and asleep)

- Watch for signs of Sleep Disordered Breathing (SDB) and underdeveloped craniofacial structures in children:
  o Mouth breathing when awake or asleep
  o Frequent ear infections
  o Dark circles under eyes
  o Snoring, noisy breathing, gasping for air when sleeping
  o Bedwetting
  o Night terrors
  o Restless sleep, restless limbs
  o Waking up groggy, grouchy
  o Behavioral issues/temper tantrums/meltdowns
  o Referrals from teachers etc. to have ADD or ADHD evaluation

If these signs are found, seek an airway-focused dentist and ENT for evaluation and sleep study if appropriate.

- Don't use a strong antimicrobial mouthwash – protect your good oral microbes.
- Do tongue scrape/brush every time you brush your teeth.
- Have your nitrate levels in your saliva checked and increase your greens or consider nitric oxide supplements.
- Adopt a breathing practice.
- Detox your household air.
- Eat oxygen-rich foods, like fruits and vegetables.

- If you have chronic allergies or sinusitis, seek help to breathe through your nose. See an airway-focused ENT or allergist such as Wyndly for information on SLIT.
- Get screened for oral signs of SDB by your dentist or dental hygienist:
  - Recession, notching at the gumline
  - Wear, flattening, chipping of teeth, erosion
  - Clenching, grinding, cracked teeth
  - Large tonsils
  - Large tongue that hides the throat when opening
  - Bony growths on the inside of the lower jaw or palate
  - Scalloping of the side of the tongue
  - Tongue or lip ties
  - Difficulty opening wide, limited opening, pain in TMJ
  - Inability to suction tongue to the roof of the mouth
  - Crowded teeth, relapsed orthodontics, permanent premolars, bicuspids removed, malocclusion
  - High vaulted, narrow palate
  - Narrow, small jaws

If you have any of these oral signs of SDB – seek an airway-focused dentist for evaluation of your airway to include a sleep study.

CHAPTER 3

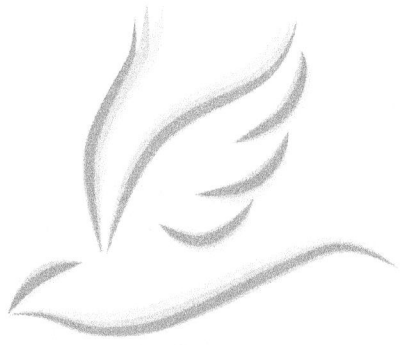

Hydrate

"Water is the driving force of all nature."
— Leonardo Da Vinci

Dehydration is a serious and potentially life-threatening problem. A few years ago, my mother gave us a big scare. She lived alone and had been sick for several days. She was nauseous, vomiting, and couldn't keep anything down, which my sisters and I didn't find out till later. She was never much of a water drinker and didn't have a very big appetite either. This was not a good combination. She hadn't been drinking anything or eating anything while she had been sick.

When my sister and I couldn't get in touch with her, we went to her house to check on her. We found her in the bathtub, semi-conscious and incoherent. Apparently, she had gotten dizzy and fell backward into the tub. She was taken to the hospital by ambulance, where she would spend the next five days. She was severely dehydrated, and her electrolytes were out of balance. Not to mention, as a type 2 diabetic, she was at high risk of going into a diabetic coma if we hadn't found her when we did. It was a very close call. It's estimated that two million people die of dehydration every year. This is a shocking statistic. *Drink water!*

After oxygen, water is the next most important need of the human body. We can survive between three and seven days without water, depending on environmental conditions, level of health, activity, and age. After seven days without water, serious health issues and possible death are imminent. The human body needs to be hydrated for many reasons. Our cells cannot perform their normal functions without water. Their structure and shape depend on water. It is a solvent and is used to transport nutrients into the cells and waste products out of the cells. It is also needed for many chemical reactions and electrolyte balance. Water is essential for saliva production and digestion.

Saliva is a buffering agent in the mouth and has many purposes and is made up of many components. Regarding hydration, water helps maintain the pH balance of saliva, which is important for preventing cavities and keeping the oral microbiome a friendly environment for commensal bacteria (good bacteria). The first step of digestion starts in the mouth with our saliva. It moistens our tissues and contains enzymes, proteins, minerals, and other important nutrients for our teeth and for our good microbes. It is actually part of our immune system. More on this later.

Water is also needed to form synovial fluid to lubricate our joints and regulate our body temperature. It maintains blood volume, blood pressure, and is crucial for cognitive function and mood regulation. And yet some people hate to drink water. This, I don't understand. It is literally the only thing I drink. I've never liked alcohol or coffee, both of which can dehydrate you.

I think it is really interesting that muscle tissue contains more water than fat tissue, hence people with higher muscle mass will have a higher percentage of water in their body. This is another good reason to increase muscle mass. Other reasons will be discussed later in Chapter 5. This is why men generally have a higher percentage of water in their body than women. Men have an average of 60% water and women have an average of 55% water. Muscle contains about 75% water while fat contains only 10% to 30%. *Amazing*!

Because muscle contains such a high percentage of water, dehydration has a negative effect on muscle function. Dana Cohen, MD, in her book *Quench*, which discusses other ways to hydrate besides drinking water, says gentle exercise like stretching that involves moving the joints helps your body maintain hydration. I'll discuss more benefits of movement in a later chapter.

Fascia, which is the fibrous collagen-based soft-tissue and extra-cellular matrix (ECM) that surrounds our muscles, organs, and other structures of the body is made up of mostly water and, interestingly, water in a gel form. Fascia is the structure that literally holds us together. Its proper function, health, and hydration is necessary for our stability, movement, performance, and recovery from injury. New research is emerging about the effects of fascia dehydration and its relationship to pain in the body. Fascia is now recognized as a biomechanical regulation system.

This neuromyofascial (nerves, muscles, and fascia) web of tissues work in concert to give us structure, stability, and the ability to move—the main function being the function of stability. Fascia, which was once overlooked by the medical world, is now considered the "organ system of stability." It touches every structure of the body from head to toe. As mentioned earlier, the fascia of the tongue can be tied in a way that restricts movement down the fascial lines (more on this later). According to Gina Bria, co-author of *Quench*, fascia needs water so that our tissues can glide over one another by keeping them wet, pliable, and elastic. It is much more complicated than this, but the basic idea is hydration is key to the health of every tissue in the body.

I mentioned water in gel form regarding fascia. Well, there is a newly identified phase of water called gel water. It is also known as structured water, living water, EZ (exclusion zone) water, and liquid crystalline water. Its molecular structure is H_3O_2, which is one water molecule (H_2O) with one extra hydrogen atom and one extra oxygen atom. It can be liquid, or thick like Jello and is highly conductive. Gel water is found in vegetables, fruits, collagen, chia seeds, and cacti. It is more easily absorbed by cells because it is charged the same as the water in cells. This is how we can "eat" our water. Aloe is a form of gel water and has various uses in health products. Dana and Gina recommend adding chia seeds to your water to help your body retain it longer as they are digested.

Adding salt or electrolytes to your water is more hydrating as well. Fortunately, proper breathing oxygenates your blood and improves the body's ability to hydrate!

I love it when we can get more than one benefit from our efforts. Because the body works so efficiently and doesn't waste anything, this is something that we will see throughout this material. There will be multiple benefits to multiple systems that can be gained from each of the foundational behaviors I discuss.

The amount of water recommended for people to drink varies from eight 8-ounce glasses per day to half of your body weight in ounces per day. There is no consensus. It depends on your level of health and activity, and the environmental temperature and humidity. Most sources agree that if you wait to drink when you are thirsty, you are already dehydrated. Suffice it to say, most people are functioning in a state of dehydration.

Keep in mind that many symptoms of illness are actually signs of dehydration. The book *Intracellular Hydration Breakthrough* by C.W. Willington, MD, goes into great detail about how hydration at the cellular level is necessary for optimal health. Prevention of chronic disease, cellular energy, mitochondrial function, and physical performance depend greatly on hydration at a cellular level. Drinking water doesn't always translate to cellular hydration. Consider the above when working on staying hydrated. Drinking water too fast or too much at once can result in more trips to the restroom and not actually hydrating our cells.

Key Points:

- Don't take drinking water for granted, it is essential for life.
- Drink at least one 8-oz glass of water immediately upon waking to replace water lost during sleep.
- Eat foods that contain a lot of water, such as cucumbers, celery, and watermelon. *Eat your water!*
- Drink bone broth for hydration, gut health, and collagen.
- Add salt, electrolytes, or chia seeds to your water to help increase cellular hydration.
- Increase the quantity of water you drink when the weather is hot and dry.
- Gently exercise, move, and stretch to help hydrate (think of yoga, but not hot yoga).
- Consider the timing. Drink first thing in the morning and before meals to maximize hydration.
- Watch for early to moderate signs of dehydration:
  o Dry mouth, lips, eyes
  o Thirst
  o Dark yellow urine
  o Lightheadedness, dizziness
  o Fatigue, headache
- Watch for signs of severe dehydration:
  o Rapid heartbeat
  o Rapid breathing
  o Extreme thirst

o   Confusion, irritability
o   Lack of sweating
o   Very dark urine

People with signs of severe dehydration need **immediate medical help** as they may go into hypovolemic shock, which is life threatening.

CHAPTER 4

Nourish

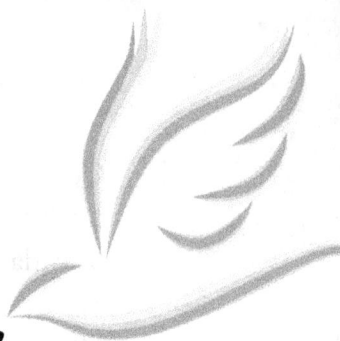

"Let food be thy medicine and medicine be thy food."
— Hippocrates

Who hasn't struggled with the issue of diet? Even if you have never been on a "diet", your diet (simply the food we eat) has a significant impact on your health or lack thereof. I am going to be fully transparent. This has been the biggest struggle in my life. Because my father was in the military, we lived abroad most of my youth on military bases. In the sixties and seventies, transportation was not as easy as it is today, especially when it comes to fresh food. Our food came mainly from the commissary (grocery store of the military), and it was highly processed, shelf stable, or frozen. Most of it was in a can or a box or a freezer. *Who remembers "TV Dinners"?* I admit I really liked them as a kid because, of course, they were loaded with excitatory chemicals. *Hmm, whose idea was that anyway?*

I hated vegetables as a kid because spinach and green beans from a can were awful. The only "vegetable" I liked from a can was corn because it was not as terrible as the other mushy stuff. I know now that corn isn't even a vege-table and that I have a sensitivity to it (the GMO strains). Our usual meal was some type of meat, a vegetable, and potatoes, rice or Stove-Top Stuffing. *Who remembers that?* We rarely ate salad and when we did have it, it was ice-berg lettuce with cucumber and carrots with low-fat or no dressing. Iceberg lettuce is not the greenest of greens. I rarely use it for salad now. My siblings and I loved cereal, graham crackers, Ritz crackers, pop tarts, and chips. With these staples in my diet, it's no wonder I had weight issues.

And if my steady diet of processed foods was not bad enough, the low-fat craze that started in the fifties, when my mom was a young woman trying to watch her figure, added to the poor choices in an effort to stay slim. Less "fat" to ward off heart disease, equated to more sugar to make the food taste better. Then there were the hydrogenated fats and margarine. It was a recipe for metabolic disaster. I started yo-yo dieting at a young age (when I wasn't even fat). It was just a thing. Girls were obsessed about their weight and there was always a new fad diet to feed their obsession (pardon the pun). We won't get into the body image aspect of the culture I grew up in, but that was a huge problem as well. I always thought I was "chubby" growing up but looking back at photos of me as a child, teen, and young adult proved I was anything but.

It amazes me how we have gotten so far from sim-ply eating healthful whole foods to nourish our bodies. Modernization, in an effort to make things more conve-nient, really made a mess of things. *Why did eating healthily get to be so hard?* It should be simple, and it really is, once you get back to the basics.

All the essential nutrients, amino acids, vitamins and minerals are available in whole foods. Yes, we know the soil is depleted from nutrients, and that organic is better than conventionally grown produce, however I would argue that eating a non-organic apple is better for your body than a candy bar, chips, or fast food. The cost of food is increasing, but so is the cost of disease management and treatment. Get the biggest nutrient bang for your buck by eliminating the ultra-processed "food" products and buy only foods that look like food or are minimally processed with NO added sugar, preservatives, chemicals, or bad fats (seed oils, canola oil, hydrogenated oils). Cutting out the junk food will save money in the short and long run.

Now, I am not a vegan or vegetarian. I do love a good steak, but I love my veggies, too, now that I don't eat them out of a can. The research from every source related to human health is pointing to a mainly "plant-based" diet. There are some health benefits from the carnivore diet as well, but I personally don't feel that it is a diet that is meant for humans long term. My reason is that in Genesis 1:29 God said, "I give you every seed-bearing plant on the face of the whole earth and every tree that has fruit with seed in it. They will be yours for food." So, per manufacturers' instructions, we are to eat plants, their seeds, and fruit for food.

The health of our gut microbiome depends on keeping our good guys fed (via prebiotics), so they can maintain the integrity of our gut lining, which keeps bad stuff out of our body. Plants provide food for our good guys mainly via their fiber content. Fiber is their fuel. And coincidently, we cannot digest this plant fiber without these microbes. They digest them via fermentation, a process that produces many of the vitamins and nutrients we need but can't produce on our own. Examples of these prebiotics (food for microbes) are inulin, resistant starches, gums, pectins, and fructooligosaccharides. When someone is experiencing a lot of gas and bloating or other gastrointestinal issues like constipation or diarrhea, it's because there is an imbalance in their gut microbiome. They don't have enough good guys to break down the fiber and this produces excess gas.

Resistant starches are interesting. One of the many "diets" I did back in the day was the Atkins/low carb diet. I stayed away from rice, bread, pasta and all kinds of starches to get my body to burn fat for fuel. A starch is basically a complex carbohydrate which, for someone who is overweight, can increase fat storage because it triggers an insulin spike which tells the body to store fat. So, the bottom line was it worked until I started eating carbs again. What I didn't know then was there were resistant starches that can't be completely digested in the small intestine (where they are absorbed as fuel). Instead, these starches pass through the small intestine to the large intestine and become food for the microbes there which produce short chain fatty acids (SCFAs) which have many health benefits. Short chain fatty acids are anti-inflammatory, and support the gut, brain, liver, and immune system.

Resistant starches have several health benefits. They are filling, due to the high fiber content. They can improve insulin sensitivity. They are helpful in reducing cholesterol, improving bowel regularity, and reducing the risk of colon cancer.

So, what constitutes a resistant starch? Barley, oats, beans, lentils, potatoes, plantains, and nuts to name a few. However, overconsumption of anything can be a bad thing. The trick with resistant starches is two-fold, eat in moderation (always a good plan for health) and then cook and cool them. Think potato salad, pasta salad, or leftover pizza or pasta eaten the next day. Cooking a starch, then cooling it down by refrigeration and reheating if needed, makes it pass through the small intestine virtually unabsorbed, thereby reducing the amount of calories you absorb by about half. I always knew I liked enchiladas better the next day. More food for thought! *I couldn't "resist!"*

In studying the microbiome and my own Biome FX stool test from Microbiome Labs, I found out that the gut microbiome ferments carbohydrates via a pathway called Saccharolytic Fermentation which is a preferred fuel for the gut microbiome and is a "clean" process that produces short-chain fatty-acids (SCFA's) that support healthy gut barrier function. It also ferments proteins via a pathway called Proteolytic Fermentation which produces SCFA's and unfavorable byproducts that are pro-inflammatory. Gut dysbiosis is associated with higher levels of Proteolytic Fermentation. Balance is key!

Many people worry about eating plants because they contain oxalates. Calcium oxalate can build up in the body in joints and in the kidneys to form kidney stones which can be very painful. Besides forming kidney stones, an excess of oxalate buildup in the body can increase inflammation and cause nerves to be overly excited, possibly leading to muscle twitching or tremors. Too much oxalate can lead to metal toxicity because metals like mercury and lead bind to them, potentially trapping them in various tissues in the body. Most people with a healthy gut microbiome can handle a reasonable amount of consumption. However, excessive oxalate consumption by someone with an unhealthy or dysbiotic gut (leaky gut) can lead to problems.

Gout is another painful joint condition. It is caused by high levels of uric acid, which crystallize in joints, most notably the big toe. Historically, high uric acid has only been linked to gout, with the major culprit taking the blame being purines. Purines are mainly found in red meat, shellfish, and organ meats. People who have gout are generally given a drug called allopurinol and told to decrease consumption of red meat. But there is more to the story. Other factors can cause increased uric acid levels, a fact that is rarely passed on to the patient. Fructose, especially in fruit juice; alcohol, mainly beer and spirits; ultra-processed foods; and excess sugar in most forms are just as responsible if not more responsible for what is driving increased levels of uric acid in the general population.

So why do these foods and drinks trigger the increased production of uric acid you ask? The answer is in David Perlmutter, MD's, book called *Drop Acid*. He not only explains why this trigger exists, but he also illuminates the impact uric acid has on chronic inflammatory disease. You see, there are other problems associated with high uric acid levels to be considered besides the link to gout. Gout is actually the lesser of two evils when it is compared to metabolic dysfunction.

High uric acid levels devastate metabolic health by signaling the body to increase fat production and deposits. This leads to obesity and diabetes. It triggers inflammation contributing to other chronic diseases such as hypertension and heart disease. It also contributes to fatigue because it impairs energy production of the mitochondria. Just like everything else that can cause us problems in our health, there are lifestyle factors that can increase uric acid levels. Poor sleep, chronic stress, and dehydration can also increase uric acid levels. So here is another thing linked to hydration. We'll talk about sleep and stress in later chapters.

I'm not going to leave you hanging on why we evolved to increase fat production and storage with the consumption of all this sugar. But it makes sense once you learn about it. Our ancestors went through times of food scarcity. During the winter, people needed a lot of fat stores to survive till spring. Think of the bear. What do they eat to fatten up for hibernation? Berries, pounds and pounds of berries. They enter a state of hyperphagia (excess hunger). *Hmm. So, eating a lot of sugar causes excess hunger?* Now it's making sense. The consumption of the abundance of fruit at the end of the summer signals the body that "winter is coming" as Dr. Perlmutter says. This increase in excess fructose, sugar, and sugar alcohols increases uric acid. The increase of uric acid signals the body to store fat. It is a survival mechanism. Only now, with our modern grocery stores and availability of all kinds of sugar all year long, we are signaling the body to increase fat deposits for a winter that never comes.

And we wonder why obesity and chronic inflammatory disease is affecting one of every two American adults and children. This is a sad and alarming statistic. Yet, every day in grocery stores across the country, well-meaning parents are filling their carts with 100% fruit juice, yogurt loaded with sugar, cereal, and sports drinks. Not to mention the other highly processed foods like chips, crackers, cookies, and snack cakes. And let's not forget the amount of fast food being consumed because of busy schedules. I know it's hard. I am guilty of eating all this stuff and feeding it to my kids when I didn't know how bad it was. But now I know better, so I am trying to do better. That is all we can do, try to make better choices every day. I believe that if people knew the long-term effects, they'd make better choices most of the time. So, education is key.

Another thing you may have heard of—and that people often worry about—are lectins. Lectins are natural toxins found in plants that help protect them from predators, such as insects. Supposedly Tom Brady, ex-quarterback of the Patriots, was on a low-lectin or lectin free diet to improve his athletic ability. Steven Gundry, MD, started the lectin-free movement when he wrote a book called *The Plant Paradox*, which talks about the dangers of lectins. In the book he also discusses how to reduce them through various cooking methods such as soaking, sprouting, pressure cooking, boiling and draining the water from greens such as spinach. Knowing how bad ultra-processed food and sugar are for you, I find it interesting that some people will actually avoid some plant-based food and choose ultra-processed foods to avoid oxalates and lectins. I think we need to see the big picture and pick our poison. Someone once said that the dose makes poison, but I can't remember where I heard that.

But I do know this: there's an ancient Greek phrase, *pan metron ariston*, which means 'everything in moderation.' It all goes back to the idea of how we were meant to eat. There were no Costcos or supermarkets in our ancestors' time. The food was scarce. People had to hunt and gather, and they eventually learned to plant gardens around their homes. The food was seasonal. They weren't able to buy pounds of spinach, chard, or beans everyday year-round. I think that the reason oxalates and lectins have been found to be detrimental to some people is because of the quantity and constancy of eating the same things that would normally not have been the case.

I don't believe that God would have told us to eat plants and fruits if they were going to harm us. I believe the normal cycle of seasonal eating and availability of food allowed the body to process and utilize what was available and keep the body in health. Food preparation was also different back then. For example, nuts and beans were soaked prior to eating or cooking. Corn was first soaked in lime water then dried and ground into flour. Cooking your own food is always a better choice when it comes to health.

A little more on the gut microbiome. In Chapter 2, I quoted Genesis 2:7 that stated, *"The Lord God formed the man from the soil of the earth."* So, as I see it, we were formed from the soil, plants grow in soil, and our gut houses trillions of bacteria that come from the soil. *Coincidence? I think not.* These microbes that make up our gut need to eat plant fiber to thrive and do their job of helping digest our food, control our immune system, and produce vitamins and hormones for our use. We are connected and dependent on the soil of the earth.

Our gut microbiome has a tremendous influence on our health and well-being. The Human Genome Project was initiated in 1990. Since then, there have been hundreds of studies and thousands of papers written about the various human microbiomes. We have more than one. We have a microbiome on our skin, in our nose, our throat, our mouth, our gut, and our reproductive and excretory areas.

The gut microbiome is connected to every system, and if not working properly, it begins to leak pathogens (bacteria, yeast, viruses, and parasites), lipopolysaccharides (LPS- toxic byproducts of microbes) and proteins into the body, setting up an autoimmune response. We know that autoimmunity is when the immune system starts attacking the body because things that aren't supposed to get into our bloodstream start "leaking" into it from an unhealthy and damaged mucous membrane. The term *leaky gut*, also known as intestinal permeability, is a chronic inflammatory condition that is associated with many inflammatory conditions such as: gastrointestinal disorders like Crohn's, IBS, liver disease, obesity, insulin resistance, fibromyalgia, chronic fatigue, arthritis, and even mental illness.

How does the gut begin to leak you may wonder? The intestines, which are basically our gut, is a one-cell-thick membrane with a layer of mucus that stands between the outside of our body and the inside of our body. Did you know that our digestive system from "tongue to tail" is actually a tube that is considered to be outside of our body but runs through our body. *What a concept! I digress.* A "leak" implies that something that is supposed to be inside a container (our gut or digestive tract) is "leaking" into the body. The leak is a gap in the tight junctions between cells of the intestinal walls. You see, the microbes in our gut need to eat. If we don't feed them the fiber, phytonutrients, polyphenols, etc., from plant-based foods, they start eating the protective mucous layer of the intestines, then the toxins they produce and the ultra-processed, pesticide-laden foods are able to poke holes in the mucous layer and pass through in a state the body can't use or recognize. Hence, a hyperactive immune response ensues.

This shouldn't happen because the digestive tract is selectively permeable, meaning it has intelligence that is supposed to only allow nutrient molecules, vitamins, minerals, and gases to pass through. It is not supposed to let toxins, microbes, or undigested proteins into the body/ bloodstream. When toxins, microbes, or unwanted substances leak into the body/bloodstream, the immune system overreacts and causes inflammation and sensitivity to these proteins that are not properly broken down before being absorbed into the body. In short, this is how autoimmunity occurs. The immune system attacks proteins from a food that isn't properly broken down and then, *voilà,* the person develops a sensitivity to that food. The food or "Frankenfood" we eat is essentially information for the body. Every molecule has information that the body needs to function properly.

There are many risk factors that contribute to the issue of leaky gut: a low-quality diet which is high in sugar and fat, and low in fiber; high consumption of alcohol; excess use of over-the-counter anti-inflammatories and antibiotics; food allergies; high stress; poor sleep; metabolic syndrome, and liver disease. Robert Lustig, MD, retired pediatric neuroendocrinologist and author of the book *Metabolical*, says to, "Eat real food," and that the two most important things a person can do for their metabolic health is to, "Feed your gut and protect your liver." Dr. Lustig also believes that sugar is harmful and one of the biggest contributors to metabolic dysfunction. *We already talked about how to feed your gut, but how does one protect their liver?*

Well, the low-hanging fruit is limiting alcohol. I am sure you have heard of cirrhosis of the liver or fatty liver disease, which used to be prevalent in mainly middle-aged male alcoholics. However, a new type of disease of the liver is on the rise. It is a non-alcoholic fatty liver disease (NAFLD), which is the same kind of destruction of the liver, without the alcohol. The cause is excessive consumption of sugar, especially in the form of fructose. Not only high fructose corn syrup, but fruit juices as well and refined sugars which are pervasive in the standard American diet (SAD).

The liver makes cholesterol, which we need, but when there are excessive amounts of sugar/fructose being consumed and needing to be processed by the liver, it has to store it in fat cells. Eventually, the liver itself starts to store the fat in and on itself, which makes it sick, sluggish and unable to do its job of detoxification. Excess sugar in any form spikes insulin which triggers fat deposition. These sugar spikes are known to damage our blood vessels and cause other inflammatory issues. Inflammation equals oxidation which equals oxidative stress which is bad for our health.

So what tools are there to help us monitor our blood sugar levels and learn how different foods affect it? Well, diabetics check their blood sugar upon waking and periodically throughout the day. However, blood sugar is fluid and constantly changing, especially in relation to when and what you consume throughout the day. Continuous glucose monitors (CGM's) are wearable glucose monitors that can monitor blood glucose around the clock, helping the wearer see how certain foods affect their blood sugar. Your primary care physician can prescribe a CGM for you if you are in a state of prediabetes or a diabetic. *But how can you be proactive and go upstream to prevent getting too close to the borderline?*

One way is an online platform called Levels Health, which provides education and coaching through the use of CGM's to help people improve their metabolic and cognitive health. Dr. Lustig and Dr. Perlmutter are medical advisors for Levels and Casey Means, MD, is one of the founders. Dr. Means has written a book called *Good Energy*, which focuses on metabolic and mitochondrial health as the foundation of health and how blood sugar control is critical for them both. She recently gave testimony in a bipartisan Senate Hearing on American Health and Nutrition: A Second Opinion. It was a four-hour discussion of the Root Cause of why Americans are sick and what to do about it with other physicians and health advocates including Senator Robert F. Kennedy Jr.

This hearing with all of its expert testimony gives me great *Hope for Health* in America and the world. It took place on September 23, 2024. You can listen to the entire replay on Dr. Means website or Rumble and read her entire testimony which lays out what she believes is behind the chronic disease epidemic we are in. She illuminates the reasons that human health is being decimated by preventable metabolic disease and states that we are not just facing a health crisis in America, but a spiritual one too. Spiritually and morally, we need to put people over profit. Dr. Means asserts that courageous leadership, smart policy, common sense, and intuition can restore the health of Americans in a couple of years because our lives and our planet are miraculous creations. It's an exciting time in history and we all need to join the fight for our very lives.

* * * * *

Now, I want to connect the health of the mouth to the rest of the body and, most importantly, the gut. We use our mouths to nourish our bodies. What we put in it matters. Like I said before, there is a lot of research being done regarding the link between the gut and disease. And the mouth is the gateway to the gut. Hippocrates said, *"Every disease begins in the gut,"* over 2000 years ago and science is proving he was right. Chronic disease, which is primarily preventable, is linked to dysfunction and dysbiosis of the gut.

So, it is worth repeating, microbes in the gut are vital to the function of our immune system. They regulate immune cell function; they produce toxins that act like antibiotics to eliminate harmful microbes and can release anti-inflammatory compounds to protect us from infection and disease. Nourishing the beneficial microbes (commensals) in our mouth and gut to promote oral and systemic health is the key to restoring, improving, and optimizing health.

As I mentioned earlier, we can nourish our commensal microbes with prebiotics. Prebiotics for both our oral and gut commensals are found in various plants that we eat. I discussed specific gut prebiotics earlier. Our oral microbiome needs similar nutrients. Xylitol, inulin, and polyphenols are some of the oral prebiotics. Several toothpastes, mouthwashes, and sprays are now being made with ingredients that feed our good oral microbes. FYGG (Feed Your Good Guys) toothpaste, which was formulated by functional dentist, Mark Burhenne, DDS, has prebiotics in it and is free of harmful ingredients that are found in most traditional toothpastes. Another company that is making dental products with the health of the oral microbiome, and non-toxic ingredients in mind is SuperMouth, which was also invented by a dentist, Kami Hoss, DDS, who is the author of *If Your Mouth Could Talk*.

Dental products that are free of toxic ingredients, balance oral pH, feed the good guys and have remineralizing properties are finally showing up in the marketplace.

Nanosilver mouthwash is one of my favorites and was also invented by a dentist, Matt Callister, DMD. It is a pH-balancing product that is plant-based and helps create an oral environment that reduces the risk for cavities, remineralizes teeth, and reduces root sensitivity.

There are around seven hundred species of microorganisms found in the oral microbiome and, just like any of the microbiomes in and on the body, some of the species are beneficial and some are not. Just like any population of living things, the good and bad need to find balance and live in harmony. Even the bad guys can serve a purpose. So, if we are too aggressive with trying to kill the bad microbes in our mouth with mouthwash or in our gut with antibiotics, or on our skin with excessive antimicrobial washes, we end up wiping out all the microbes, even the good ones that we need. This potentially results in bad side effects like leaky gut, and/or an increase in the opportunistic bad guys.

The oral microbes that are the most hazardous to our health and put us at high risk for chronic disease are: Aggregatibacter actinomycetesmycomitans (Aa), Porphyromonas gingivalis (Pg), Treponema denticola (Td), Tannerella forsythia (Tf), and Fusobacterium nucleatum (Fn). These are the top five high risk pathogens. They are vascularly aggressive and are present in periodontal disease. Once they are established in high numbers, they can enter the bloodstream and translocate to other organs and systems, wreaking havoc in their wake.

So how do we get these bad microbes you ask? Well, all the microbes in our microbiomes come from our family and our environment. Babies get their first exposures from their mother through the birth canal and from touching her skin, nursing and from putting their little hands in their mom's mouth and then in theirs. I know it sounds gross, but we know that babies always have their hands in their mouths, and they touch everything. This is critical to establishing their own immunity. It is by design. Children whose parents are germophobic and overuse antimicrobials inhibit the child's immune system. Many of these children develop allergies and sensitivities and get sick easier because their immune system was not adequately challenged as a baby. If grandma or grandpa had gum disease or any of these pathogens and they shared their spoon with the baby or cleaned their pacifier with their own mouth after it fell on the floor, which I have seen, they just inoculated that baby with their oral microbes.

Research shows us that Aa is linked to cardiovascular disease, stroke, brain abscesses, and heart infections to name a few. Pg is considered a high-risk factor for heart attacks, strokes, rheumatoid arthritis, dementia, and Alzheimer's disease, among others. Td is a spirochete that is very hard to get rid of and is linked to dementia and Alzheimer's. Tf and Fn are also linked to these inflammatory diseases and Fn is also linked to colorectal cancer and adverse pregnancy outcomes.

These and other pathogens can be identified with salivary testing. There are several companies that are doing salivary testing of various kinds. Two such companies I have worked with are Simply Perio, which is a DNA PCR test that tests for twelve microbes and four viruses.

Another test I run for slightly different information is the Bristle test. It is a shotgun genomic test that looks at the whole oral microbiome and all the species present. It evaluates different risk factors based on the whole population. For example, it gives scores for risk for cavities, risk for gum inflammation, and risk for gut inflammation, as well as gives scores for a number of beneficial bacteria and number of nitrate-reducing bacteria that help make nitric oxide. As dental professionals, with the information from these salivary tests, we are able to indentify the pathogens, treat the mouth to help restore homeostasis and lower the risk of chronic disease. *This is huge!* I don't understand why every dental office is not offering this to their patients. *This needs to change.* In my mobile practice, I test every patient as part of their initial appointment and then follow-up as needed to see the changes achieved from treatment and behavior modifications.

Most people don't know the link between oral pathogens and systemic disease. Sadly, not enough of my fellow dental professionals are focusing on educating their patients about it. If I had a nickel for every patient that says, they have never been told this information, I'd have a nice little vacation fund. In my experience, when they do learn about it, they feel empowered and onboard to do something about it. When given the information and education, I find that most people want to do what they can to improve their health. We need to give our patients more credit than we do.

If your dental professional is not offering this test, let them know you are interested in doing it to find out not only your risk for periodontal disease, but the risk for the systemic diseases associated as well. More of these tests are being offered directly to the consumer because more and more people are interested in taking ownership of their health and want to optimize it. Taking advantage of the technology available is wise. *Why should we keep guessing when it comes to treatment of gum disease and managing chronic disease, when we can test for the pathogens responsible so we can treat them with a targeted approach?*

Treatment can consist of laser assisted non-surgical periodontal therapy; targeted antimicrobial treatment delivered in custom trays, like hydrogen peroxide gel in Perio Protect trays; irrigation with antimicrobial liquids, gels, or ozone gas; desiccation therapy; oral prebiotics and postbiotics; gut prebiotics and postbiotics and, of course, improved home care.

Antibiotics can also be used with discretion. It is not my first line of treatment because we don't want to wipe out the good guys along with the bad. This causes other problems, not to mention the overuse of antibiotics causing resistant strains of microbes. However, in certain instances antibiotics are needed if the patient is at high enough risk for a life-threatening event.

For example, I had a patient who was only thirty-eight years old who had suffered a stroke only nine months prior to my testing his oral microbiome. He had high numbers of Aa and Pg as well as Td and Tf. Given he already had a stroke recently and the oral pathogens likely contributed to it, we decided to target the Aa and Pg with an antibiotic and support his gut microbiome with gut probiotics and prebiotics. Post testing three months later showed that the Aa and Pg were eliminated and the Td and Tf were also greatly reduced. Through improved homecare on his part, taking oral and gut probiotics and increasing prebiotics, he continued to bring balance to both the oral and gut microbiomes.

When trying to increase the foods that feed the good guys (prebiotics), consider adding garlic, onions, leeks, asparagus, bananas, artichokes, berries, apples, citrus fruits, grapes, kiwi, green tea, cocoa, dark chocolate, oats, barley, carrots, mushrooms, and legumes. These foods are considered health foods mainly because they feed our gut microbes and therefore improve our health. It's strange that we didn't really "know" this till recently. It's slowly becoming common knowledge with the advent of the internet and social media, but unfortunately it isn't widely known enough, because we still have an avalanche of chronic disease and it's extremely difficult to convince people to shift from ultra-processed foods and eat whole foods instead.

Many people find it hard to increase plant-based foods. It requires more frequent trips to the grocery store for fresh produce, lots of preparation, washing, chopping and then cooking. Let's face it, many of us have schedules that are so busy, it's hard to manage to eat healthy consistently. Thankfully, we can cheat a little and still get our healthy greens, phytonutrients, fiber, etc. with organic super green powders that you can add to water and drink as a high nutrient shot or it can be added to smoothies or soups. One of my favorites is Power for Life Superior Greenfood Plus by TerraOceana. It has it all, phytonutrients, antioxidants and probiotics. Even if your diet is pretty good, these types of dietary supplements can fill the gaps and give you the added boost you need to help nourish, detoxify and enhance your immune system.

An exciting emerging novel technology created by Emily Stein PhD is Selective Microbial Metabolic Regulation Technology (SMMRT™). It applies nutrient pressure to the oral microbiome with prebiotic and post-biotics that in essence block carbohydrate metabolism by the oral microbes, ultimately reducing the pathogens like Pg and increasing the beneficial bacteria. It also balances the pH in the mouth. The overall result is a health promoting oral microbiome. This has very promising potential for improved oral and systemic health outcomes.

We know that the macro nutrients needed for the human diet are proteins, carbohydrates, and fats. Of the three, protein is the most important building block in the human body. However, worldwide, it is estimated that over one billion people are deficient in this nutrient, and it is also estimated that fifty percent of homebound elderly are significantly deficient as well. Being protein deficient is probably the reason they are homebound. As we age, we need more protein for protein synthesis for both mechanical and structural purposes. The best source of protein is animal protein because it has all the essential amino acids. It is a complete protein, which means it has all the essential amino acids. Plant proteins can be a good source of protein, but they are incomplete proteins containing some of the essential amino acids. Because plant proteins are incomplete, they need to be combined with other plant proteins to form complete proteins. This can be accomplished with a little research and imagination. An example is beans and rice, which is a staple in many cultures. Individually, they are incomplete in the 9 essential amino acids, but together they have a full compliment.

There is a lot of controversy when it comes to eating animals as it relates to cruelty and the environment. When it comes to the environment, vegans cite concerns about deforestation, greenhouse gas emissions, water usage, and land degradation in animal agriculture. This is true of industrial farming practices; however, science is proving that sustainable and regenerative animal farming practices can be environmentally beneficial. Our ancestors practiced sustainable and regenerative practices naturally. Modern industrial practices are responsible for the environmental woes of the planet not our ancestral sustainable and regenerative practices.

The argument between vegans and non-vegans is multifaceted, involving ethical, environmental, health, cultural, and economic viewpoints. However, as highlighted in the documentary *Need to Grow*, the planetary destruction of our nutrient-rich soil by industrial farming is leading to a threat to our food security worldwide. Nutrient-rich soil is composed of essential minerals (both macro- and micronutrients), organic matter, beneficial microorganisms, proper soil structure, adequate moisture, air, and a suitable pH level. It is a balanced ecosystem where plants can thrive, and roots can grow. The nutrients in the soil that are needed for the plants to grow are the same ones we need to grow. *Need to Grow* stresses the need for regenerative agriculture and sustainable food practices or we may not have any healthy soil to grow our food in by the year 2073. Again, this is food for thought (pardon the pun), very important food for thought, but not the subject of this book.

So back to the subject of protein. I never knew the importance of protein, or the amount required to keep me healthy. I have learned that the recommended daily allowances for food and the food pyramid I grew up with are not adequate and are much lower than what is needed for optimal health. Prioritizing protein to build and maintain muscle mass is key. Sadly, most of us consume far less protein than we need for optimal health.

According to Gabrielle Lyon, MD, author of *Forever Strong*, and other experts on muscle-centric health, we need a minimum of about one gram of protein for every pound of ideal body weight. Most people are deficient in protein. This deficiency causes a weakened immune system, bone and muscle loss, edema (swelling), and skin and hair changes.

I admit that getting enough protein has always been a challenge for me. Dr. Lyon asserts that we need a minimum of thirty grams of protein per meal to initiate protein synthesis. How many people eat two eggs for breakfast thinking they are getting enough protein? I did. Two eggs is only twelve grams of protein. Adding a healthy yogurt with low or no sugar can get another 18 to 20 grams. *She says we need a minimum of ninety grams per day!* But it can be done with intention and planning. It can seem difficult because it was for me, but for vegans, it's even harder because they need to eat a lot more volume to get that amount of protein. It is much easier to do by combining animal protein and plant protein together and the plants are better for your gut microbiome. However you slice it, the fact remains, consuming enough protein every day is extremely important if you want to optimize your health and health span.

There are so many nutrients in whole foods. This is why we need a variety. William Li, MD, wrote a great book called *Eating to Beat Disease*. The book talks about the different nutrients in different foods and the effects on the body of various foods. I like how he lays everything out in tables and lists. He describes the various foods needed for the Five Health Defense Systems and the foods that support them. These Health Defense Systems are: Angiogenesis (building of blood vessels), Regeneration (making of new cells), Microbiome, DNA protection, and Immunity. Another great book about eating for health is called the *Dental Diet* by Steven Lin, DDS. He looks at food not only based on nutrient needs but also on functional needs, like hard foods being necessary for optimal growth of the craniofacial (head and face) structure.

The EWG (Environmental Working Group) has a Clean Fifteen list of the top fifteen non-organic produce that have the least amount of pesticides and toxins. The 2024 Clean Fifteen are carrots, sweet potatoes, mangos, mushrooms, watermelon, cabbage, kiwi, honeydew, asparagus, sweet peas, papaya, onions, pineapple, sweet corn, and avocados. So, not all produce needs to be organic to be healthy. This is money saving. They also have a Dirty Dozen list of produce that has the most pesticides and toxins. The Dirty Dozen in 2024 are strawberries, spinach, kale, grapes, peaches, pears, nectarines, apples, bell and hot peppers, cherries, blueberries, and green beans. They recommend you buy organic products on this list to reduce the toxic burden on your body. There are nice graphics available to download that have pictures of both of these lists. I recommend printing them out and laminating them to put on your refrigerator or to take with you when you go grocery shopping.

While there are many foods that have health benefits, not every person responds well to every food. Again, bio-individuality comes into play. It's not that a particular food is unhealthy for a certain individual, but that the individual may be sensitive to certain foods because of their particular health condition, especially their gut health. Gut dysbiosis is responsible for many things that ail us. *Remember what Hippocrates said about all diseases starting in the gut?* This puts many people in a pickle because it is hard to find out what foods are beneficial for whom. A superfood for one person may give another person the runs. *So, what is one to do?*

Have hope! The health of your gut microbiome can be determined by working with a functional health practitioner that can order a stool test to see who's living in there and what to do if it is dysbiotic (out of balance). Microbiome Labs has a stool test called Biome FX. It also has spore-based probiotics and protocols to get things back in balance and restore your gut to health. A direct-to-consumer company called Viome has a Total Body Intelligence test that tests blood, stool, and saliva to give you personalized health recommendations.

I did the Viome Gut Microbiome stool test in 2019, and found out the foods that are superfoods for my microbiome and foods I should avoid and why. The idea is that you avoid the foods that are harming your gut and eat the foods that will help your gut heal; then retest in six months to a year (or sooner) to see if your gut is healing and tolerating foods that were on your avoid list. Ideally, we should be able to eat all foods in moderation if our gut is healthy as it was created to be. Diversity of the gut microbiome is considered healthy and this diversity comes with a diversity of food choices. Most people eat as little as twenty to thirty different foods day after day. Considering the variety of food options there are, that number is pretty low.

Consider herbs for seasoning food, there are over 300. There are over 1000 vegetables cultivated in the world and 2000 fruits. Then there are around 21 different grains, and 23,000 different types of legumes! *Wow!* But animal protein is the most diverse. There are literally millions of different species of living things that can be eaten, from carnivores, herbivores, to omnivores, mammals, fowl, fish, shellfish, mollusks, fungi, insects, reptiles, and the list goes on. *We need to do better!* (Personally, I'll probably pass on the insects and reptiles, although I heard alligator and snake taste pretty good.) Look in your refrigerator and pantry and see what you can do to increase the number of herbs, spices, fruits, and vegetables you can try. Step outside of your box and comfort zone. Be adventurous. You might find some new things you like.

So, when it comes to food allergies and sensitivities, I am not discounting that there are exceptions, like those that have Celiac Disease and other diseases. Work with your health practitioner when trying to figure this out. There is so much we can do to improve our health and wellness when it comes to our diet. It just takes some imagination, courage, and exploration.

It is worth it though. Diet plays a huge role in health. Every chronic illness stems, in some way, from a dietary issue. I used to think that if I ate something that tasted good, but was not good for me, I could just do a little more exercise and it would balance out. I know people who say I work out so I can eat what I want to, meaning junk food, sweets, or alcohol. However, someone once told me that you can't out-exercise a poor diet. Diet is a part of the foundation of health that will make or break us.

Like I said earlier, we can send a message to the food producers of unhealthy ultra-processed foods, by boycotting so-called "foods" that contain:

Additives: "natural" flavor, emulsifiers, thickeners, anti-foaming agents, dyes, artificial sweeteners, and sugar

Oils: seed oils, hydrogenated oils, chemically produced oils

Preservatives: propionic acid, butylated hydroxyanisole (BHA), monosodium glutamate (MSG),

sulfur dioxide, potassium benzoate

This list is not comprehensive, but a good rule of thumb is that if there are more than three-to-five ingredients listed on the label, and you can't pronounce them, or it's in a shelf-stable package, chances are you shouldn't be eating it.

* * * * *

Lastly, when it comes to eating, it goes without saying that most of us eat too much, too frequently, and with too little variety of whole foods. The subject of eating too much is being addressed by many health advocates, with a practice that has been around for millennia. The practice of fasting is one you may have heard of. Fasting has been practiced for religious reasons, health reasons, and when food was scarce. The practice of fasting crosses many cultures and traditions. Fasting is thought to have many benefits physically, mentally and spiritually. Since we are talking about the body, I'll point out the physical benefits.

Autophagy and cellular repair take place while we are fasting, usually while we sleep. Autophagy is when the body is triggered to clean up dead or dying cells and make new ones. Detoxification of the body is also ramped up during fasting. Because digestion is a very energy-intensive process. When digestion isn't happening, the body can use the energy to detoxify and get rid of dead cells and waste. This is what is meant when we say that the body is resting and repairing during sleep.

It is obvious that we aren't eating when we sleep, so this process generally happens when we sleep. However, it is believed that autophagy and cellular repair can happen any time that we are not eating for an extended period of time. However, it works best when the time of fasting is longer than just the eight or so hours we sleep. Intermittent fasting has become a popular practice for people trying to optimize their health. The term intermittent means you are fasting for longer periods of time beyond when you sleep to gain health benefits. It can mean skipping breakfast, skipping lunch or skipping dinner. There are many ways to do intermittent fasting. Valter Longo, a biochemist who has deeply studied the health benefits of fasting, created a fasting-mimicking diet that can give you the same benefits of fasting called Prolon. It has prepackaged fasting "meals" where you get to eat while fasting. If you want more information to learn more about how fasting helps your health, read *The Complete Guide to Fasting* by Jason Fung, MD. While working with patients with kidney failure due to diabetes, he found that fasting was the best way to help them control their insulin, blood sugar and help them lose weight. His mantra is that anyone can do it, and everyone can afford to do it because it is free. You don't have to buy pills or special meals, or special foods and it will save you money while helping you get healthier.

People are realizing that overeating, eating too frequently, and eating food that is of little nutritional value is leading to obesity, metabolic health issues, and chronic disease. The other benefits of intermittent fasting are improving metabolic functions such as insulin sensitivity and supporting weight management. Fasting promotes fat burning by using up stored glucose and switching to burning ketones for fuel. This switching back and forth between burning glucose and burning ketones is called metabolic flexibility. It is an innate survival mechanism that our ancestors went through in times of food abundance and food scarcity. The problem now is that there is an abundance of food and people eat constantly during every waking hour without giving their systems (liver, kidneys, intestines, etc.) a break.

Inflammation is part of our innate survival mechanism as well. All inflammation is not bad. Inflammation is needed to protect us from opportunistic bacterial infections and viruses. It is an integral part of our immune system. It heals our wounds. The problem is chronic inflammation, which occurs when our body is overwhelmed by toxins, sugar, and overwork. Our body is a hard-working machine 24/7, but certain systems need a break to rest and repair. Fasting gives the body the time that it needs. It actually reduces inflammatory markers.

One of the best benefits is regarding the brain. When we fast, there is an increase in brain-derived neurotrophic factor (BDNF). BDNF supports cognitive function and is thought to protect against cognitive decline and neurodegenerative disease. Everything points to fasting having a myriad of health, mental and spiritual benefits, and I think we could all benefit from skipping a meal now and then. However, fasting isn't appropriate for everyone. People with certain health conditions (e.g., diabetes, eating disorders, or pregnancy) should consult their healthcare provider before beginning a fasting regimen and when appropriate fast with the support and monitoring of their health provider.

Key Points:

- Test your oral and gut microbiome annually to improve health, they can be remodeled.
- Remember the top five Pathogens that are linked to systemic disease Aa, Pg, Td, Tf, Fn.
- Remember food is information to our body; don't feed it misinformation.
- Eat whole foods, as much organic as possible.
- Remember the Clean Fifteen and Dirty Dozen.
- Eat a variety of every type of food.
- Don't be afraid to try new foods.
- The more colorful the fruits and vegetables are, the more nutrient-rich they are.
- Feed your good guys in the mouth and gut with dietary prebiotics.
- Protect your liver by limiting alcohol and pharmocologics, if possible.
- Prioritize protein even if you are vegetarian or vegan.
- Eat thirty grams of protein per serving/meal to assure protein synthesis.
- Try to extend the period of time you are not eating between dinner and breakfast. Even a few hours will help your digestion and organ resting.
- Stop eating three hours before going to bed. This benefits your digestion and sleep.
- Modulate your oral microbiome with prebiotics and postbiotics in Protektin by Primal Health LLC.

CHAPTER 5

Move

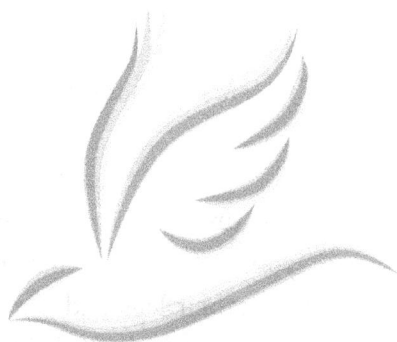

*"Exercise not only delays actual death
but also prevents both cognitive and physical decline
better than any other intervention."*
— Peter Attia

We don't move as much as our ancestors did, and it is to our detriment. Movement is essential for life. A sperm has to swim to unite with an egg, which has to travel from an ovary to the uterus. Once they unite, cells start dividing to create the thirty-seven trillion cells that make up a human. Electrical signals from our brain move through neurons to the rest of the body to control everything from breathing to initiating our bodies' movements. Our blood moves from our heart to the rest of our body through the movement of heart muscles. Lymph fluid relies on the movement of our diaphragm when we breathe and movement of our feet and legs, since it has no pump of its own. If we don't move, our lymphatic system can't balance our fluid levels, remove toxins, or send out white blood cells to attack viral and bacterial invaders in our bloodstream.

Even before we were born, we moved and kicked. Just ask any woman who carried a child in their womb. Have you ever noticed that infants, when lying on their backs, kick their legs and move their arms? They are training to build strength in their muscles to roll over. Every movement of their head, neck, arms, and legs is to build strength to achieve their next milestone. They roll over, sit on their own, crawl, and eventually walk and run. Once they start running, they never stop.

My grandchildren never stop moving. My grandsons are forever jumping, running, skipping, climbing, and wrestling with each other. My granddaughter, an aspiring gymnast, is flipping on the trampoline, doing cartwheels down the sidewalk, and leaping through the air at every turn. They never sit still. But this is normal, children are growing and are meant to move and stimulate their muscles, organs, and brains. And no, it is not ADD or ADHD (that's another topic). Next time you are out and about, observe the constant movement in children. My mother watches them and says I wish I could bottle their energy. They are firing on all cylinders.

What happens to us as we age and take on the responsibilities of life? We slow down, and we stop moving. We start adulting and we sit down to work, watch TV, and drive from here to there. We stop living a life of activity. According to Dr. Peter Attia in his book *Outlive: The Science & Art of Longevity, "The best predictors of a long and healthy life are mobility, strength, and balance."* People are losing these things, not because they are aging, they are aging because they aren't intentionally practicing movements that keep them mobile, flexible and strong.

Like me, he believes that simple sustainable practices are free or low cost, citing regular strength and mobility exercises, improving cardiovascular health, and mindful nourishment as methods to improve health outcomes. Focusing on simple key practices discussed in these chapters will help you foster a positive balanced pursuit of health. Awareness is key.

Something I never knew about muscle is that it helps control our glucose levels. Every contraction of your muscles is burning glucose. Atrophy (the loss of muscle) due to a sedentary lifestyle leads to insulin resistance, which eventually leads to diabetes and other chronic diseases of inflammation. Muscle is a very metabolically active tissue. The good news is that it is possible to regain muscle after it is lost, but as we age, it gets harder and harder. As we lose muscle mass our fat deposits increase. *But there is hope! It is never too late!*

Sure, starting earlier is better, but thanks to the adaptability of the miraculous machine we call our body, we can maintain and even rebuild muscle at any age. A lack of balance is the main cause for falls in the elderly, which can be fatal. Balance and stability activities are things we need to focus on as we age.

One of the reasons people are losing their ability to balance is because of footwear. You may have heard of the barefoot movement or minimalist footwear. Footwear has dampened the sensitivity of the plantar proprioceptors on the bottom of our feet. The information these sensory nerves control how our body reacts to our movement. Our feet control our movement though a deeply integrated neuromuscular system of nerves, fascia, muscles, and joints. The foot has 26 bones, 33 joints, 19 muscles and 107 ligaments. This body part with 33 joints was designed for movement of those joints.

Emily Splichal, MD, is a functional podiatrist who wrote a book called *Barefoot Strong*. Her goal for the book is to teach lifelong mobility and strength through the feet. She says, *"The foot is the gateway to our ability to experience the joy of movement."* Through foot release and foot strengthening exercises she *"empowers patients with the skills needed to maintain and restore movement at any age."* Reading her book generated hope in me that my chronic knee pain could improve because the *"feet are the foundation of all closed chain movements."* By strengthening my feet through barefoot activation, and foot-to-core integration, I believe I can be barefoot strong to improve my overall health and mobility. *I have hope!*

We talked about fascia in the chapter on hydration and its importance in the stability of our frame and movement. Stretching is important to keep muscles loose. Tai chi, yoga, and Pilates are good for balance and stability. Even things as simple as standing on one leg or walking heel-toe, heel-toe. Remember, the lack of movement of a muscle leads to atrophy (wasting away). *SO, MOVE!*

There are many ways to increase your movement in your day. Taking the stairs and parking at the far end of the parking lot to get more steps in are the low-hanging fruit. Dr. Peter Attia talks about five things we need to train for and be able to do in the last decade of our life, hopefully as a healthy centenarian.

1. Hike a mile and a half on a hilly trail.
2. Get up off the floor using a maximum of one arm for support.
3. Pick up a thirty-pound child from the floor.
4. Carry two five-pound bags of groceries for five blocks.
5. Lift a twenty-pound suitcase into the overhead compartment of a plane.

I personally want to be able to do all of these things and train for them. Getting up off the floor with a maximum of one arm for support is the biggie for me. Admittedly, my job for the last forty-five years has been sedentary. I have enjoyed exercising on and off over the years. I love dancing and used to Jazzercize a lot. I also love water fitness classes, but I need to up my strength training. The main thing is to find ways to incorporate more movement into our everyday lives and find an activity we enjoy and perhaps can enjoy with a loved one or friend so that the time passes quicker and there is opportunity for connection.

My water fitness classes have multiple benefits. I sing along with the music and socialize with my friends, which improves my mood, my cognition, and memory. It brings me joy to connect with my friends. We help each other improve our health because we hold each other accountable. We miss the interaction and the feeling of getting in a good workout when we miss a day. Knowing that I'll be seeing my friends when I go to class motivates me to go even if I don't feel like it. Once I'm there I am so glad I went. The health benefits are priceless. I am raising my heart rate and heart rate variability, increasing my circulation, engaging my brain, and improving my mental and emotional state.

What about people who have health issues or are immobile for some reason? Maybe they are recovering from an injury and have limited mobility. *Good news!* We can do isometric exercises anyplace and anytime. It is still helpful. It may not build muscle, but contracting muscles even isometrically can keep them from wasting away. Contracting them also helps lower blood sugar. Muscles release "hope molecules" (aka myokines) every time muscles contract. They are called hope molecules because these myokines are small proteins that can regulate mood, reduce anxiety and trauma, among other things. Kelly McGonigal, PhD, says *"Movement is how your brain knows you're alive and engaged in life."* Hope molecules can improve learning, protect the brain, reduce inflammation, and even combat cancer. *I love that they are called hope molecules!* Kelly also wrote a book called *Yoga for Pain Relief* and one called *The Joy of Movement.* There are so many benefits to movement.

There are many other benefits of isometric exercise. They can improve your posture, endurance, and range of motion. Additionally, isometric exercises can strengthen your bones and connective tissue (ligaments, tendons, fascia). The pull of muscles on bones actually makes them stronger. Isometric exercise can help lower blood pressure as well.

An example of isometric exercise is to tense all the muscles in your body while lying in bed before you even get up in the morning. When you are sitting at work, or on the couch, you can work your calves by doing calf raises, leg extensions, bicep curls, or tricep kickbacks without weights, just contracting your muscles. An exercise I learned in physical therapy for my knee is quad sets, which is just contracting your quad muscles isometrically and holding for five to ten seconds. Isometric exercises can also help relieve pain.

One of the best isometric exercises you can do is a plank. It uses practically all your muscle groups. This one is not easy, and it takes some strength, so it might not be one for anyone who is injured or immobile, but planks build core stability, which is very important for our movement longevity. If you can't start with a full plank on the floor, start out by doing it on a wall and working your way down to the couch or a bench and then to the floor. Another benefit of isometrics is that they reinforce muscle activation patterns, especially after an injury or surgery. Pumping our ankles while lying in bed or sitting (especially on a plane) can increase circulation, which can prevent blood clots.

So basically, we have no excuse not to move. We are all guilty of saying we don't have enough time to exercise, but where there is a will, there is always a way! The big picture is that our efforts and movements today will pay dividends in the future.

Key Points:

- Don't stop moving.
- Get creative and find ways to move and use your muscles throughout the day.
- Prioritize muscle building and maintenance through resistance training.
- Isometric contraction of the muscles can be done anywhere, anytime.
- Find an activity you enjoy and recruit your friends and loved ones.
- Eat enough protein to build muscle, at least thirty grams per meal.
- Start training for your Centenarian Decathlon.

MIND

CHAPTER 6

Think

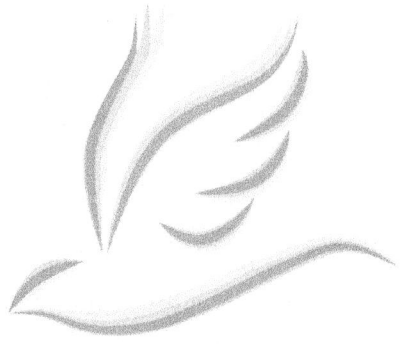

"For as a man thinketh in his heart, so is he."
Proverbs 23:7

Our minds are powerful things. Our thoughts create our beliefs and reality. The things we think about, whether positive or negative, are reality to our mind. Our beliefs and thoughts are formed as early as when we are in the womb. You have heard of expectant mothers that read or play classical music for their unborn babies during pregnancy. As early as in utero, the human brain is being influenced by the sounds around them. There is a phenomenon coined the Mozart Effect relating to classical music being played for babies still in the womb to increase their IQ. While much of the evidence of this is anecdotal, there is evidence that infants develop an affinity for music and voices they heard while in the womb.

Similarly, a mother's emotions during pregnancy can greatly affect the unborn child. The fetus is exposed to and affected by the chemical and hormonal signals that are released with various emotions of the mother, both positive and negative. Stress and anxiety can negatively impact the unborn baby's growth and development. It can also affect their neurological development, which could possibly lead to mental disorders like autism. It is also thought that it can influence its temperament.

If a woman is fearful or traumatized during pregnancy, the fetus can have anxiety and even experience the trauma the mother did. Our environment and the things we sense or hear during every stage of our life get recorded and are a basis for our beliefs. Emotions are powerful and the spoken word is very powerful too. God spoke all of creation into existence. He gave us free will and the power to choose our words. *"Death and life are in the power of the tongue."* Proverbs 18:21.

I grew up saying, *"Sticks and stones may break my bones, but words will never hurt me."* But that was a lie. Words do hurt and can play in our minds over and over. We know that bullying can cause long-term damage to the receiver and can lead to mental health issues and in some cases suicide. *Words are so powerful!* Negative words we speak to ourselves are particularly harmful. Negative thoughts we have about ourselves are known as negative self-talk. These thoughts can be conscious or subconscious. The great thing is that positive thoughts or affirmations can cancel negative thoughts. The Bible says, *"Whatever is true, whatever is honorable, whatever is just, whatever is pure, whatever is lovely, whatever is commendable, if there is any excellence, if there is anything worthy of praise, think about these things."* Proverbs 4:8.

What we believe and say to ourselves and others is so important. People talk about manifesting things into their lives and the law of attraction. I believe that because God created us in His image, and he spoke the universe into existence, that our words also have the same power to manifest in our lives the things we speak and believe. This goes for the good and the bad. When we believe negative things, they are called self-limiting beliefs. My friend Michelle Prince (also my publisher) wrote an inspiring book called *Shine Through Your Story*. She put it this way, *"Whatever your beliefs are, you're putting actions and behaviors in place around those beliefs."* So, we need to speak and act on the positive things in our lives, not the negative.

We are all guilty of berating ourselves at one time or another, but there is hope! God thought of everything! Romans 12:12 says that we can *"renew our minds."* We can change our thinking and change the pathways in our brains. We now know that the brain has neuroplasticity. Caroline Leaf, PhD, author of *Switch on Your Brain*, explains that neuroplasticity means, *"Our thoughts, emotions, and experiences can reshape the very structure of our brains, allowing it to adapt and change over time."* Another example of how our beliefs can influence our bodies is something we have all heard of called "the placebo effect." This occurs when someone is given a 'sugar pill' and told it will have an effect on their body— and, lo and behold, it does, simply because they believe it will. No matter how you look at it, the mind is incredibly powerful!

Understanding the power of the mind can change everything. The possibilities are endless. God wants us to live in abundance. Jesus said that he came to give us an abundant life in John 10:10. That means abundant health too. Deuteronomy 30:19 says, *"I have set before you this day life and death, blessing and cursing therefore choose life that both you and your descendants may live."* The life we live is up to us to choose.

What thoughts and beliefs are holding you back from living the life you dream of and the health you wish for? I challenge you to reflect on the thoughts that keep you from living your abundant life. Write them down and rewrite an affirming statement that cancels that thought. Mindfulness is a buzzword that is used a lot these days. Be mindful of what you say to yourself and others.

I have been challenged with weight issues and knee pain. My limiting beliefs were that I would always struggle with my weight because of my genetics and that bad knees run in my family. Now I say that I am able to achieve and maintain an optimal weight to support abundant health and that my knees are healing and will function perfectly the way God intended. Romans 14:7 says that God calls things that are not as though they are. I take this to mean that whatever we are believing God for in our lives, that we will have it if we believe and speak it into existence (eventually). It's not magic, hocus pocus, or instantaneous; sometimes it takes patience and work on our part to see it manifest in our lives, but we must have faith and never lose hope. This doesn't mean believing you will win the lottery will make it happen, and it doesn't mean that challenges in our health, finances and relationships won't happen. *They will.* It's more about having the things that are God's will for our life, such as love, peace, joy, and health. I personally believe that having and keeping faith, hope, and love are the keys to happiness and contentment in this life.

Keeping a positive attitude about all of life's circumstances and giving people the benefit of the doubt is beneficial not only for your peace of mind, but for your health too. Remember, your attitude toward life and circumstances is based on what you think. Perspective is everything. *Is your glass half full or half empty?* Most challenges and obstacles in life can be opportunities for change or growth depending on how you look at them.

Key Points:

- Understand that what you think day in, and day out consciously or subconsciously has power over your life.
- Make a conscious effort to speak positively to yourself and to those around you.
- Know that what comes out of your mouth (your words) affects the rest of your body.
- Try to have an attitude and perspective that obstacles and setbacks are opportunities.
- Remember you have the power to overcome adversity.
- Reflect on your negative beliefs and reconceptualize them into positive affirmations.

CHAPTER 7

Grow

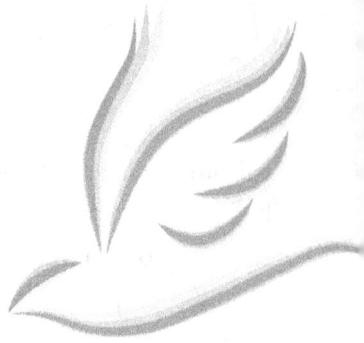

"Growth is the only evidence of life."
— John Henry Newman

Every living thing starts out as a seed or a single cell. In the cycle of life, we are in a state of growth to a certain point, some say between twenty-one and thirty-ish, and then we start to die, some of us faster than others. It all depends on epigenetics. *What are we doing to promote health or promote a quicker death?* The growth of our bodies is one aspect of growth. This is considered our physical growth, but what about our intellectual, emotional and behavioral growth?

Our intellectual growth is considered to increase with age. We often call this wisdom. Cumulative knowledge and experience have traditionally been valued in our elders. *Is this still true of our modern-day culture?* Eastern cultures are more respectful of the elderly and value their wisdom more than Western culture. However, this is a generalization and varies depending on a family's traditions and beliefs. I believe that with the rise in cognitive decline due to poor diets and lifestyles, the elderly are losing respect because they are thought to be losing their mental capacity because of age, irrespective of their health status.

This is a sad reality that can be turned around. Our aging population can improve their cognitive ability with diet, exercise, and continued learning. You have heard the phrase, *"Use it or lose it."* This is true not only for muscles as we discussed in Chapter 5, but also for the brain. Of course, it is better to start sooner than later and be proactive about all things health related.

When people retire and stop using their brain to solve problems and learn new things, it starts to atrophy. We are fortunate that there are many resources online to improve cognitive function. However, simple things like reading, dancing, singing, playing an instrument, exercising, and activities with coordinated movements make a big difference in cognitive function. I am a lifelong learner and believe that learning new things will keep the mind sharp. Doing crossword puzzles, playing cards, or other board games are other ways to use the brain, so you don't lose it. My favorite game to play with my grandkids is *Match Madness.* Everyone gets a set of five blocks that have colors and shapes on four sides that are used to replicate a pattern on a card that has one of five different levels of difficulty. The winner is the one who replicates the pattern first. *It's really fun!*

Emotionally, we grow through life experiences. The areas of emotional growth are in our ability to manage ourselves. Being able to regulate our emotions, thoughts, and behaviors and taking responsibility for our actions demonstrate our emotional growth. Having self-awareness, empathy, and social awareness are also aspects of emotional growth. People who lack these abilities can seek counseling or take personal development courses to improve in these areas.

When it comes to behavior, there is always room for improvement. After all, none of us do the right thing all the time. We fall off the wagon with eating healthy, flossing our teeth, and practicing mindfulness, to name a few. So, in the area of behavior, the opportunities for growth are endless. This book highlights many areas where we can change behaviors to improve our health. As we know, behavior is a hard thing to change without effort. Change in behavior has to become a habit. There are many books on the topic of habits, you may have heard of the book *Atomic Habits* by James Clear and perhaps the practice of habit stacking. I like habit stacking, because if you have already established a habit of doing one thing, you can stack another thing onto that habit and, by associating a new habit with an established habit, you develop a new habit.

My favorite habit stack to help my patients is regarding flossing. Most of them brush twice a day. So, what I tell them to do to establish the habit of flossing, is to floss first at night before they brush, that way they won't skip the flossing. If they continue to brush first, it's too easy to skip the flossing like they are in the habit of doing. *You see how that works?*

Having a growth mindset is when you see everything as an opportunity for growth. Setbacks and obstacles are important for growth and improvement. Embracing change is an aspect of growth. Focus, persistence, patience, curiosity, and open-mindedness are characteristics that help people grow personally and professionally. Growth keeps us from becoming stagnant and lifeless. Stagnation leads to decline, decay, and death. We must keep growing in every area of life. Learning and experiencing new things is the spice of life. Don't be afraid of learning or trying something new.

Key Points:

- Remember that growth is necessary in every stage of life.
- Your cognitive function is a use-it-or-lose-it function.
- Continue to use your brain in a variety of ways to stay sharp.
- Personal development and professional development courses, programs. and books are good investments for your well-being.
- Find ways to adopt new behaviors that serve your health and well-being.
- Try new things.
- Keep learning.
- Stay curious.

CHAPTER 8

Create

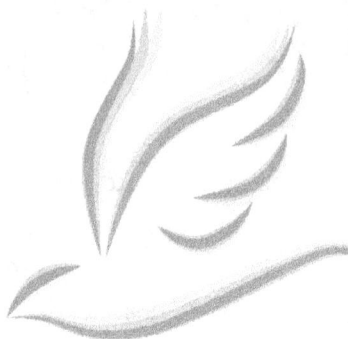

"When we move toward our own creativity,
we move toward our creator."
— Julie Cameron

I have always loved to create things. One of my favorite things to do when my girls were growing up was to make their costumes for Halloween or plays at school. I loved using glitter, different colored paints and materials. *Oh, what I could do with a glue gun!* The girls were always so thrilled with them and after the event they were intended for, they would add them to their "dress-up" bin. Now that they have kids of their own, I still help with costumes when I can and am the official face painter for all their birthday parties.

I love the imagination of children. I remember in the summer when the girls were home for summer break and as a single mom, I couldn't afford to take them on nice vacations like their friends. So, they would make up plays, make up dance routines, and occasionally bake some cookies or a cake and decorate them. They'd leave their chores to the last few minutes before I got home, but I loved seeing their latest artistic creations.

Our creator created us in their image. Therefore, I believe we are "Wired to Create." According to authors Scott Barry Kaufman and Carolyn Gregoire, children use play to understand themselves and their environment. Have you ever noticed that when small children open a gift for their birthday or Christmas, they somehow end up having more fun playing with the wrapping paper or box more than the contents? Kids can have a room full of toys and use pillows, chairs, and blankets in the room to build a fort. They love to build and create things with whatever is in their environment. I think this is why my grandkids love Legos so much.

Art is a creative expression. Dancing, singing, painting, cooking, or creating a craft is all an outlet for a gift that God gave us. He created this beautiful planet and created everything that lives and breathes. Can you imagine the imagination it took to create giraffes, pandas, parrots, flowers, and fruits, to name just a few of His creations? *Amazing!*

These days, creativity is evolving to include content creators for blogs and videos for social media. Innovations in technology and industry are another form of creativity. Did you ever play make believe or build a fort or play cops and robbers when you were a kid? Did you dream of inventing something? Or draw plans for your dream house? Creativity sent men into space and put them on the moon.

Creativity helps us solve problems and think outside the box. It's where invention is born. Do you remember exploring when you were a kid? When we lived in the Philippines, there was a golf course near our house that had a big jungle area next to it. There was a sign that said "Danger! Keep Out!" on a big chain across the entrance, but that sparked our imagination even more. There was a stream running through and dense foliage all around. We would "pan for gold" in the stream and walk barefoot through the tangled vines that we pretended were snakes we had to jump over. Thinking back on it, there were probably snakes hiding in there somewhere, not to mention unexploded ordinances (also something I learned later); hence, the "Danger! Keep Out!" sign. We were a bunch of carefree kids with an attitude of positivity that gave us the confidence to wander the jungle with abandon.

Being creative boosts your self-confidence and well-being. It gives us the opportunity to look at things from a different perspective. It can be a way to reduce stress and make you more able to adapt to different environments and situations. Some people might think they aren't very creative, but we all have some measure of creativity. The world would not be where it is without all the gifts each one of us possesses. A car mechanic might think they're not creative because they can't paint or draw, but the ability to understand how things work, diagnose issues, take them apart, and put them back together is a form of creativity.

The very existence of the human race depends on our ability to create other little humans. Life goes on and has the potential to get better because of creativity and innovation. Businesses rely on creativity and innovation to survive and grow. Creativity solves problems, improves products, and productivity. Creativity is not only for the arts. New ideas are a creative outlet as well. Creativity contributes to an individual's growth and development. Like in the previous chapter on growth, a lack of creativity can bring stagnation, lack of progress, and eventually obsolescence. A person or society that doesn't progress eventually ceases to exist.

The expression "the lights are on, but nobody is home" or they are just "going through the motions" or they are "stuck in a rut" depicts someone who has ceased to grow or create. Again, I will say that the mind is a powerful thing. But the mind has to choose to engage in life. It's a matter of deciding to live and grow and create. Taking action can be both hard and easy—it all depends on perspective. What's harder: doing nothing or trying something new? Personally, I have the mindset of 'so much to do, so little time.' I take advantage of all the creatives out in the world who are sharing their creativity through the internet. I want to learn and try everything.

I wake up every day wondering what I can learn and how I can help. Life is more fun, exciting and enjoyable with a creative mindset. Jeff and Staney DeGraff said, *"Creativity can make ordinary people do extraordinary things!"* in their book *The Creative Mindset*. Life is what you make it! Use your imagination and have fun! YOLO!

Key points:

- Try new things.
- Use your imagination.
- Don't let yourself get stuck in a rut.
- If you do, take action to get out.
- Create the life you want.
- Dance like no one is watching.

CHAPTER 9

Sleep

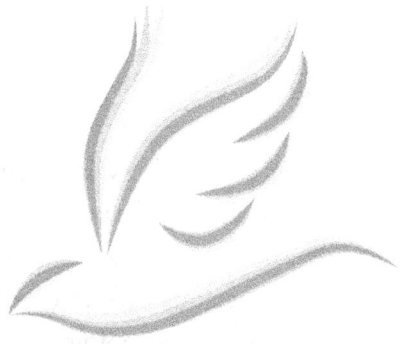

"A well spent day brings happy sleep."
— Leonardo Da Vinci

Do you remember a time when you thought sleep was a waste of time? When kids are having fun and it's time for bed, they don't want to go to sleep. Bedtime is often a stressful time for many families. As I remember it, trying to get the girls to bed when they were tired but were fighting the sleep because they didn't want to miss out on anything was utterly exhausting. Kids don't understand the important benefits of sleep. They just know they don't want to stop playing.

Taking naps was another time of contention between mom and child. As adults we wish we could take a nap. We know when we are tired and when we long for the peace that comes when your head hits the pillow. However, modern life has interfered with our normal sleep cycles. We used to wake up at sunrise and sleep once the sun set. With the advent of the lightbulb, our workdays got longer, and our sleep time got shorter. It's almost a badge of honor to declare how little sleep one gets. Sleep deprivation is widespread. Even in children.

In *Sleep Wrecked Kids*, Sharon Moore discusses the deleterious effects of sleep deprivation on children. Kids might be sleeping, but their sleep quality is insufficient. Many children are sleep deprived due to airway issues, which can be seen such as snoring, mouth breathing, restless sleep, and bedwetting. However, consequences that are easily overlooked because they aren't typically associated with sleep deprivation are developmental challenges, health challenges, as well as emotional and behavioral challenges.

Developmental challenges in sleep-deprived children include trouble with memory, concentration, and problem solving. Speech and language can be delayed. Grouchy, anxious, stressed, and irritable children can be experiencing a lack of restful and restorative sleep. Some symptoms of sleep deprivation can mimic ADD or ADHD. Things like impulsivity, aggression, and difficulty regulating emotions—you know, "melt downs" over the smallest things. Some children may be on medications for ADHD that are actually suffering from sleep deprivation. So, the root cause of the problem is not being solved, and the long-term effects can be chronic disease in adulthood or sooner. Obesity, reduced immune function, and impaired growth are also potential consequences of sleep deprivation.

These little ones need our help. We need to raise awareness of this issue. Do a better job of screening for the medical or dental root cause such as nasal allergies or obstruction and tongue ties or misaligned teeth due to underdevelopment of their face and jaws. Identification, treatment, and support for children and families suffering from these correctable issues takes education and collaboration between the various health professionals. Like I said before, it takes a team to support and restore a person's health.

In general, sleep is taken for granted and not made a priority. I know that when I was a single mom in college with four little girls, I was lucky if I got four hours a night. In his book *Why We Sleep*, Mathew Walker illuminates the importance of sleep. Sleep is finally getting recognized as a necessity, not a luxury. Our very lives, health, and well-being depend on our quantity and quality of sleep. Thanks to science, we now know that many very important functions take place in the brain and body while we sleep.

I only recently heard of the glymphatic system. It is the lymphatic system of the brain. It removes toxins and waste from the brain as we sleep, especially when we sleep on our side. The most important substance the glymphatic removes is beta-amyloid. Beta-amyloid plaques in the brain are believed to contribute to Alzheimer's dementia. It's amazing that something as simple as restful sleep can help prevent cognitive decline.

Why is good sleep so elusive? Longer work schedules, electronic devices, artificial light, some medications, disruption of hormones by environmental toxins, caffeine too close to bed, as well as alcohol before bed are all sleep disruptors. The biggest offender linked to poor sleep is the invention of the lightbulb. But more specifically, modern lightbulbs that are more energy efficient but are not emitting the full spectrum of light and are mostly emitting blue light that is very stimulating to our retina.

Light suppresses the production of melatonin, which is a hormone that causes us to get sleepy. This affects our circadian rhythm (the body's normal twenty-four-hour sleep and wake cycle). God is so clever. Our innate function revolves around the rising and setting of the sun, which has been disrupted by artificial light. Melatonin is suppressed when our retina is exposed to light and it is activated when the retina does not have light stimulation (when it is dark).

Given this phenomenon that light suppresses melatonin and dark increases melatonin, wearing sunglasses may affect melatonin production by increasing it during the day which may induce sleepiness. Also, light increases serotonin levels. Serotonin is the feel-good hormone that improves mood and it also is a precursor to melatonin. If there isn't enough light exposure in the eyes to produce serotonin then melatonin is also inhibited. So, reducing light to the eyes via sunglasses, may have the potential to have the same effect on people that get seasonal depression when sunlight is limited in the winter. This is something to think about. I don't know, would God have created eyes that couldn't handle the sunlight that lights our days? I personally have never worn sunglasses. I can go out in bright sunlight and not have to squint, which a lot of people find odd. I get a lot of exposure to sunlight in my eyes, and I am generally always in a good mood. Maybe there is a link.

There is a new term known as sleep hygiene. You may have heard of it. It involves creating a sleep-friendly environment to promote healthful sleep. This includes creating a dark room with no sources of light that can be detected by your eyes even when your eyes are closed. Room temperature is also important. It should be very cool, around 65-69 degrees. Keeping electronics out of the bedroom is also recommended and staying off of electronics thirty minutes before going to bed. One should also stop eating three hours before going to bed and maintain a consistent sleep schedule. Getting natural light early in the morning and at dusk helps to regulate our natural sleep cycle. Ideally, we should sleep seven to nine hours.

There are two main sleep cycles, REM and non-REM. During non-REM sleep, the body is resting and repairing. It is the physically restorative part of sleep. It is a state of deep sleep where memories are consolidated. REM sleep is a cycle with rapid eye movement. In this cycle of sleep, dreaming, emotional regulation, creativity, and problem solving can occur. Poor sleep can have a negative effect on mental health by contributing to depression and anxiety. Sleep apnea is associated with increased anxiety as well.

The health benefits of good sleep include, better cognitive function, better metabolism, better weight management, better cardiovascular health, better immune and mental health, and better relationships. Conversely, sleep deprivation impairs cognitive function, leads to obesity and diabetes, cardiovascular disease, and a weakened immune system. And of course, as I previously discussed in Chapter 2, adequate oxygen is needed during sleep to achieve the maximum health benefits.

Family dynamics and relationships can be greatly affected when children and or their parents aren't getting enough sleep. No one benefits when parents or kids are tired and grumpy. It puts stress and strain on the whole family. Maybe you have been there. I know I have. But there is hope for healthier sleep if you make an effort to implement these key principles.

Key Points:

- Be proactive about identifying sleep issues with children as early as possible.
- If symptoms of poor sleep are seen, have their airway evaluated.
- Evaluate your own sleep habits.
- Set an example for children by exercising sleep hygiene:
    o Have a consistent sleep schedule.
    o Power off electronics at least thirty minutes before bedtime.
    o Switch to full spectrum lightbulbs in lights you use after dark to reduce blue light.
    o Get natural light from the sun in the early morning and at dusk.
    o Keep the bedroom temperature cool (65-69 degrees).
    o Keep the room as dark as possible, use black out curtains, and remove anything with a light.
    o If a child needs a night light, use a red light which doesn't affect melatonin levels much.

- o Refrain from eating at least three hours before bedtime.
- Set yourself and your family up for successful sleep by creating sleep-friendly environments for all.
- Prioritize sleep for everyone in the family.

SPIRIT

CHAPTER 10

Love

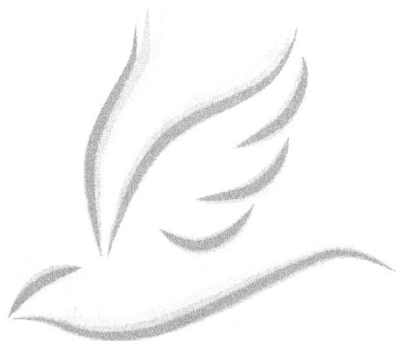

"Let all you do be done in love."
1 Corinthians 16:14

Love is a basic human need. It is a strong human emotion but is much more than that. It is multifaceted. In the Greek language, the different types of love have different words. There is a word for erotic love, unconditional love (like God's love), mature love, familial love, affectionate love, obsessive love, playful love, and self-love. I think the English language misuses and overuses the word love, and I am guilty of it. People say they love a social media post, or they love coffee. I have been known to say, *"I love these shoes!"*

However, I believe that love, in its deepest meaning, is pure and requires action. Love seeks to benefit others. 1 John 4: 7-8 says "Beloved, let us love one another, for love is of God; and everyone who loves is born of God and knows God. He who does not love does not know God, for God is love." John 3:16 says "For God so loved the world that He gave His only Son, that whoever believes in him shall not perish but have eternal life." Then Jesus said, "This is My commandment, that you love one another as I have loved you." in John 15:12. The word love is used over three hundred times in the bible.

Can you guess what the most common theme of music is according to a psychology of music study? *Yup! You guessed it, LOVE!* Since 1960, sixty-seven percent of songs are about love. Another study found this percentage to be true in almost every decade. Love is said to be a universal language. It connects people.

Psychologists believe love plays a significant role in human survival. Anna Machin, an evolutionary anthropologist who wrote *Why We Love,* explains that love is *"as fundamental to us as the food we eat and the air we breathe."* I remember learning about children in orphanages that didn't get love or affection, who failed to thrive and often died. 1 Corinthians 13:13 says, "Three things will last forever—faith, hope, and love—and the greatest of these is love." It is the love of humanity that feeds the homeless and brings relief to war-torn countries or communities affected by natural disasters. Our deepest instinct is to love one another and cooperate for our survival as a species. Love has the power to unite people with differences for a common purpose.

Each of us have gifts and talents that God gave us to serve one another. We cannot survive on our own. We need each other. The Bible says that we are one body that relies on each of the parts doing their share to keep the body growing and thriving. Serving one another and caring for one another expresses love for humanity. This love is what causes a person passing by a car accident to stop and put themselves in harm's way to help a total stranger. It is the reason someone would run into a burning building to save a child trapped inside. I could think of a thousand examples of someone helping a total stranger, even if doing so would put them in danger. This is love in action. It is universal love. The kind of love that drives people who go into healthcare, because they have a love for their fellow man. They want to help heal the world.

So now I will use the word *"love"* to describe how I feel about my calling and mission in life. I believe God called me into the field of dentistry when I was sixteen years old to share His unconditional love and hope with the people who come to me for help with their oral health. I am so thankful and blessed that as the years have passed, I have become more passionate about how I can help them optimize their systemic health by improving their oral health. I feel it is a privilege and honor to serve God by serving my patients to the best of my ability because I love them as God loves them.

I do my best to walk in faith every day, because of the love God has placed in me and because I believe in the reason he put me on Earth. My mission is to give hope to my patients that achieving and maintaining health and well-being is possible. And I do what I can to support them on their journey. Many people that come to me have real fear of dentistry and it is not their favorite place to be. When people are afraid, they might appear to have a bad attitude or be in a bad mood or even closed off. It's these people that need extra care and attention. They need to feel safe, heard, and understood, which can be a way of loving them.

Health in the body can only take place if it has what it needs. Love is one of those needs. This book talks about all the things that we need for health and wellness in body, mind, and spirit. We can't experience true health if any of them are lacking. If we love and are loved we can experience physical, mental, and spiritual health and well-being.

Although love can sometimes defy logic or explanation, it often has transformative power. Love can inspire forgiveness, compassion, and empathy. It can inspire change, growth, and help us overcome fear and insecurity.

1st Corinthians 13:4-8 says, "Love is patient, and kind; it does not envy or boast; it is not arrogant or rude. It does not dishonor others, it is not self-seeking, it is not easily angered, it keeps no record of wrongs. It does not delight in evil but rejoices in the truth. It always protects, always trusts, always hopes, always perseveres. Love never fails."

In 1965, when I was two years old, Burt Bacharach composed one of my favorite melodies of all time. The lyrics by Hal David were very timely when our country was at war in Vietnam. But I think the song is timeless. These are the lyrics.

"What the world needs now is love, sweet love,
It's the only thing that there's just too little of.
What the world needs now is love, sweet love,
No, not just for some, but for everyone."

Love is an endless currency that we can never run out of. It is a renewable resource that multiplies the more we give. Yet looking at our world, it is hard to believe that something we can freely give to each other is so scarce. If you look at crime, war, poverty, sickness, mental illness, and the state of our environment, you will conclude that there is a shortage of love in the world.

However, I assert that there is not a shortage of love. There is a surplus of love of self more than others, which is manifested as greed, materialism, fear of lack, hatred, apathy, indifference, and ignorance. Love of self is not bad unless it overrides the manifestations of love in 1st Corinthians 3:4-8. We must love ourselves in order to love others, but just like too much of a good thing is bad, so is love of self.

This is easy to illustrate if you are a parent. If you had a choice between you having a terminal illness or your child having a terminal illness, would you trade places with them? I don't know a parent who wouldn't. Here is another example. A plane crashes and the survivors work together to help each other survive. They help each other build shelter from the elements. They ration food and water so they can all eat. We are one body. The human race is "a" people, we are a community working together to survive on this planet.

Do you remember the famous phrase from the Three Musketeers? *"All for one and one for all!"* Unfortunately, this is not a shared value by everyone on the planet or we wouldn't have all the bad things happening that are destroying our planet and us. Cooperation is love in action.

A population working together to the same end can do anything. In the chapter on nourishing the body, I talked briefly about what is behind the chronic disease pandemic. Ultimately, there is a spiritual battle between greed and the greater good.

I believe greed comes from insecurity and fear of scarcity. Corporations are entities, run by people who are driven by the need for wealth, power, and position. The unwillingness to share resources and wealth comes from a lack of compassion and empathy. When people view their needs as more important than others, an imbalance occurs in the circle of life. Some people view the obsession with wealth and power as a trait that stems from feelings of inadequacy, self-worth, and insecurity. An article in *Social Cognitive and Affective Neuroscience* written by Wei et al., 2022, found that greedy personality traits lead to negative emotions, unhappiness, a feeling of never having enough, and an overall dissatisfaction of life. Remember the saying, "Money can't buy happiness"? I think it's true, and maybe the saying, "Money can't buy me love," like the Beatles wrote, is also true.

Living a life that embodies love is walking in a spirit of gratitude and appreciation for the connection, safety, and trust we have in one another. Love being one of the fruits of the spirit is something that is lived out in our actions and how we show up for ourselves and for others.

Ideal or true love is not possessive or conditional. It is a gift that should be freely given and have no expectation of being reciprocated. However, love is a spiritual concept that is somewhat subjective to the person who is experiencing it on the giving or receiving end. So key points and tips may be biased by my personal opinions. The bottom line is that the human experience is experienced most completely and fully when experiencing it with love at its core. As Maya Angelou beautifully said, *"Love recognizes no barriers. It jumps hurdles, leaps fences, penetrates walls to arrive at its destination full of hope."*

Key Points:

- You can't pour from an empty cup; you must love yourself to be able to love others.
- Walk out your life with an attitude of gratitude and love.
- Love is an action, not just a feeling.
- Love is an intentional effort to care, show kindness.
- Love is found in the simple joys of life.
- Love celebrates life through good times and bad.
- Love is not a fair-weather friend; it is a commitment.

CHAPTER 11

Connect

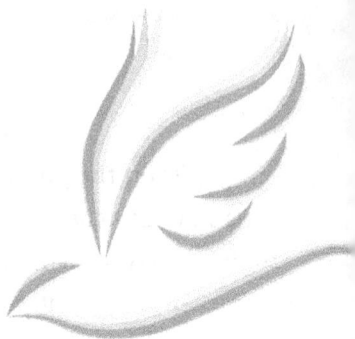

"The Lord God said it is not good for man to be alone."
Genesis 2:18

God created man to be in relationship/connected to Him. Taking time to pray and praise God for everything you are grateful for is a way to connect to Him. Reading His word is another way. God created woman because man needed a suitable partner to be in relationship with and through that connection the rest of the human race came into being. Relationship is connection. Our first connection is with God who created us. Then we are connected to our families and then to the rest of mankind. Connection to other humans is essential for health and well-being. Other health benefits of connection are reducing stress and anxiety, improving self-esteem, and boosting mood. It is also believed that connection can increase one's longevity. As a health professional, my favorite part of my job is connecting with my patients.

I have always enjoyed doing group fitness classes. I used to do aerobics classes and Jazzercise classes and now

I enjoy aqua fitness classes at my neighborhood recreation center. The best part is the social aspect. There is music, movement, and connection. We visit while we exercise and often connect outside of class for lunches or outings. Some of the women play mahjong together, which is great for their cognitive function. We support each other and care for each other, and we will all be healthier for it, not just because of the physical activity, but the connection. Our hearts long to connect with each other. Brené Brown says, *"Connection is why we're here. We are hardwired to connect with others. It's what gives purpose and meaning to our lives, and without it there is suffering."*

Because we are so dependent on connecting, there are many songs that talk about connection and being there for one another. In 1966, The Four Tops released a song called "Reach Out and I'll Be There." Here is one of the verses, *"Now if you feel that you can't go on,*

because all of your hope is gone, and your life is filled with much confusion, until happiness is just an illusion, and your world around is crumblin' down...reach out...and I'll be there." Knowing someone cares and will be there when you need them is the essence of faith, hope and love. Things we need as much as the air we breathe.

Having good social connections can offer support and accountability when needed. Social connection can bring us joy, happiness, and fulfillment. Knowing that we have people that care for us and depend on us can give us a sense of purpose. Having a purpose gives life meaning. It also imparts a sense of accomplishment and of making a difference. Kelly McGonigal says, *"Caring for others trig-*

gers the biology of courage and creates hope." Loneliness is the opposite of connection and therefore has the opposite outcome. Loneliness brings depression, anxiety, and hopelessness. Find a group of likeminded people who share your interests and see how your joy and zest for life improves.

If you haven't seen the documentary with Dan Buettner called *Live to 100: The Secrets of the Blue Zones* on Netflix, you are missing wonderful insight and hope for a longer healthier life. One of the major factors that contributes to the longevity in the Blue Zones is connection or community. Having a connection to people that support each other in times of celebration or in times of need is comforting and an essential part of the human experience.

People that belong to a faith-based community are more likely to live longer and healthier lives. A sense of belonging in any type of community has the same effect. Volunteering or being in service to others is also beneficial to your health, especially your mental health. Loving your neighbor in this way is fulfilling a purpose that is innate in humans.

There is another connection that I never thought about before, which is also very important. It's the connection with yourself. Connection with yourself is loving yourself, knowing yourself, and understanding yourself. It is also self-acceptance. Accepting yourself with all your faults and imperfections is unconditional love. It's how we should love one another, but also how we should love ourselves. This goes back to the self-talk we discussed in Chapter 6. Speak to yourself like you would speak to your child or how you wish someone would speak to you.

Remember that your words have the power to heal or hurt. Self-care and self-compassion are important aspects of connecting with yourself. One of the purposes of this book is to illuminate all the major areas of self-care.

God and man are not the only things we can connect with. Since we were made from the soil of the earth, and our body consists of all the elements of earth (mostly oxygen, carbon, and hydrogen), we need to connect with the earth. Again, modern living has taken that away from us. We have lost our connection to nature and to the earth to an asphalt jungle.

Do you remember the song "Big Yellow Taxi" by Joni Mitchell? She wrote this song in 1970. Here are some of the lyrics, *"They paved paradise and put up a parking lot. Don't it always seem to go, that you don't know what you've got till it's gone... They paved paradise and put up a parking lot."* The song also talks about putting trees in a tree museum and charging to see them, as well as farmers putting away their DDT and leaving the birds and bees. I think the message is still relevant today, maybe even more so.

I recently heard of a term called Earth Overshoot Day. It was shocking. In simple terms, it is a day in the year when consumption of resources on earth exceeds the planet's biocapacity to replenish resources and absorb waste and emissions. In 1970, when Joni Mitchell wrote "Big Yellow Taxi", Earth Overshoot Day was December 30th, when the planet was only one day in the red. In 2024, Earth Overshoot Day was August 1st. From August 2nd to December 31st, we were living on future resources. And so, it goes on, year after year, unless we change. This is an unbelievably sobering thought. It's definitely something to think about.

So back to connecting with the earth and why we should do it. Our ancestors were in constant connection with the earth. The earth has a natural negative electrical charge and when we contact it (soil, sand, grass, ocean, streams) with our bare skin (feet, hands, or body), free electrons enter our body and can act as an antioxidant potentially neutralizing free radicals. I never knew this before, but I find it so fascinating.

With the advent of insulated shoes, building materials, and sleeping off the ground, we lost our connection with these free electrons. Our ancestors wore leather footwear and slept on the ground for millennia. I remember visiting my great-grandmother who lived on a ranch in New Mexico when I was around ten years old. She had no electricity, a wood stove, kerosene lanterns, and a dirt floor. This was about 1973. I think she was nearly one hundred years old and still rode a horse, shot rabbits for food, and pumped her water from a well.

If you haven't heard of grounding, or earthing as some call it, you may think this is a joke, but a 2015 article in the *Journal of Inflammation Research* stated that, "The disconnection from the Earth may be an important, insidious, and overlooked contribution to physiological dysfunction and to the alarming global rise in non-communicable, inflammatory-related chronic diseases." It also says that "the earth's surface is a battery for all planetary life, and electrons from the Earth may in fact be the best antioxidants, with zero negative secondary effects, because our body evolved to use them over eons of physical contact with the ground." In a nutshell, the researchers who wrote this article think that chronic disease is an electron deficiency that can be reversed by simply walking barefoot and connecting to the earth.

Because many of the functions of our body are based on electrical impulses and the earth has an electrical charge, I believe connection to the earth is necessary for life. Without these electrical impulses that are generated by the movement of ions across cell membranes, our muscles couldn't contract for our movement, our heart could not beat to pump blood and oxygen to our organs, and our brain could not function to give us the ability to think and have memory. I find this so fascinating. The human body is a good conductor of energy, so we can easily absorb free electrons from the earth.

I don't understand quantum physics, but on an atomic and subatomic level, every living thing is made up of matter (protons, neutrons and electrons) and energy. Everything from water, the earth, and all its resources, and even we humans are made of the elements in and on our planet. I believe this is why we are all connected. It's why when you are thinking of someone, they suddenly call. I think things like coincidences, six degrees of separation, and serendipity are manifestations of our connection with each other on a quantum level.

If you want to learn more about grounding, watch the documentary called *The Earthing Movie* on Netflix. It talks about all the benefits and the science behind it. I personally ground for at least thirty minutes a day when the weather is nice. I walk barefoot in the grass as often as possible and lay in the grass in my backyard, enjoy nature and look for animals in the clouds. It reminds me of being a kid who can't resist rolling down a grassy hill or doing cartwheels and somersaults in a field. *(Remember this image for the next chapter.)* I have also started using grounding sheets on my bed. My husband swears his sore back from golf is no longer an issue since we started using them. I feel more rested and sleep better on them. Various companies sell them, and you can get them on Amazon as well.

There is one more thing we have lost our connection with. The natural light of the sun is essential for life on earth. Again, our modern way of life has disconnected us from the sun's life-giving energy. We live and work indoors and sun exposure has been vilified because of the potential of excess exposure and sunburn leading to cancer. I learned that we have different receptors in our eyes and skin that respond to the different spectrums of light from Dr. Alexis Cowan, who specializes in mitochondrial medicine, metabolic physiology, and light biology. Even though she knows how things work down to the metabolites being produced by different microbes in the gut, etc., she really focuses on getting back to nature. She says we weren't meant to know all the minute details, but to trust in the divine order of things. Her premise is that our natural way of living ancestrally gives us everything our body needs.

Her biggest interest and focus is light, specifically light from the sun. She talks about how the research of different light spectrums illuminates how important sunlight is to our health and all the ways it functions relative to the healthy function of our body. Light is intricately tied to our neurochemistry (the chemical messages in our bodies that control things).

Supreme Court Justice Louis Brandeis said, "*sunlight is the best disinfectant.*" Historically, people used the light of the sun and fresh air to disinfect their clothes and bedding outside. My grandmother and mother used to hang our clothes on the clothesline outside. I remember how good they smelled. Not only did they hang their clothes, but they would hang the rugs out and beat them with the broom to get the dust out of them. UVC light is known to be highly antimicrobial. It can be applied to acute wound infections to kill pathogens, especially antibiotic-resistant ones. UVC is widely applied for sterilization of inanimate objects in hospitals.

UV light exposure has been used as a treatment for psoriasis, acne, jaundice and eczema. Photo biomodulation is a new modality of light therapy for promoting healing and stimulating the immune system. Red light therapy is used for pain relief and upregulation of the immune system as well as stimulating collagen. Growth factors are released from epidermal cells exposed to UV light. Infrared and near infrared saunas are widely used for their health benefits. I use light in the form a diode laser to kill pathogens around the gums prior to cleaning my patients' teeth and when treating periodontal disease. Many of the pathogens I discussed earlier are targeted by the spectrum of light emitted from this laser.

Again, the circadian rhythm is the body's master clock. It tells the body what time it is based on light. The reason this is so important is because the clock controls the production of hormones, secretions like stomach acid, digestive enzymes and determines when they are released according to the time of day. With our modern environments the body's clock is out of sync because it doesn't know what time of day it is because of artificial light and a lack of darkness. Light pollution is not only polluting the night sky, but also our sleep and optimal bodily functions.

The benefits of sunlight go beyond the production of vitamin D. Different spectrums of light can be leveraged to improve our circadian rhythm, affecting our sleep, our mood, our stress levels, our coping mechanisms, our digestion, and can even help us lose weight. Again, I am not delving into all the granular mechanisms. Let's focus on the big picture. Knowing the importance of connecting with sunlight, and the ground is enough to improve your life and health without having to know exactly how it works. Not knowing how something works doesn't negate the fact that it works that way.

If you remember back to the basic science we learned in school, we learned about different natural laws, like the law of physics, etc. The earth, our environment, and our bodies were created with certain laws of how they function naturally. Everything will work as it should if we get back to the simplicity of the natural way of things. All the foundations of health and wellness are at our disposal.

One last philosophical thought to consider is that the reason light is important to us is that we are light beings. In my belief system, we were created by God in His image. The Bible refers to God as the Light of the World. In the military I learned about the use of *night vision goggles*. Night vision goggles allow us to see a "heat signature" which is seen in the form of light emanating from every living creature. It is known as bioluminescence.

This light emanating from our bodies can be photographed with special cameras. The picture is known as a thermogram. A thermogram is a colorful picture of the infrared energy being given off by a living body. The colors vary depending on the temperature of the surface area. It is basically a heat map of the body. One of the markers for inflammation is heat, so very hot areas in the body may identify areas of inflammation. It is a lot more complicated, but my point is that we emit light.

People often use the expression, *"They are so full of light,"* when talking about someone's energy or spirit. This figure of speech refers to positivity, optimism, happiness, goodwill, and love. People with this light radiate a sense of brightness and hope to all those around them. We need more of this light in the world.

Key Points:

- Connect with God or whatever you believe in as a higher power than you.
- Connect with yourself and learn to listen to your body and what it needs.
- Connect with others.
- Connect with the earth and all nature has to offer (hug a tree).

- Connect with the light inside you.
- Connect with the sun, especially early in the morning and before sunset. This will help you sleep.
- Get as much sunlight on your skin as you can every day, but don't burn. Use caution.

CHAPTER 12

Play

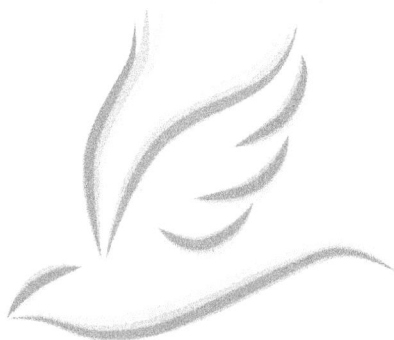

*"We don't stop playing because we grow old;
we grow old because we stop playing."*
— George Bernard Shaw

Do you have that friend or family member that is just plain fun to be around? Science says that being funny is an attractive quality and that humor is a sign of intelligence. People love to laugh. Laughing is good for the soul and releases endorphins. I especially love laughing and playing with my grandchildren. It's not just good for my soul, but it's also good for my health.

When was the last time you played? I don't mean a competitive sport, but a free unencumbered time spent without purpose. Like rolling down a hill or cartwheeling down the sidewalk or climbing a tree? Have you had any fun just for the sake of fun? I agree with George Bernard Shaw, we do start getting old when we stop playing. Why do we stop playing though? We often use the term "adulting" when we reach the age of eighteen, and we use the term "child-ish" as a derogatory term. It's no wonder as responsibility increases, that play becomes a low priority. It's become a social norm.

*   *   *   *   *

We stop playing as the pressure of everyday life and the pursuit of success increases. Then these pressures lead to stress. Chronic stress plays a major role in the development of chronic disease. Certain stressors are beneficial. There is eustress (positive stress) and there is distress (no explanation needed). We tend to think all stress is the same (negative). You ask, how can stress be positive? Well, for example, stress on our muscles helps build them, makes them stronger and helps strengthen our bones. However, this requires rest and recovery to actually complete the task of repairing or building.

The term hormesis refers to a moderate stressor that can cause cells to adapt to that stressor which ultimately improves its ability to handle more severe challenges. You may have heard of cold plunges or the use of saunas. These are examples of ways to apply the phenomenon of hormesis. These types of things make us more adaptable and can be fun and even a game of challenge you play with yourself! High-intensity interval training (HIT) is also a type of exercise that works this way.

Another somewhat positive or beneficial type of stress is one that motivates you to take on or complete a task or goal, learn a new skill or sport, or take a risk like riding a roller coaster or going sky diving. It can bring about a feeling of excitement or eagerness. The key is that this type of stress is short-term and can often enhance focus and performance. Think of the feeling of having to make a speech or meet your significant other's family for the first time. Kelly McGonigal explains why stress can be good for you in her book *The Upside of Stress.*

*　　*　　*　　*　　*

Stuart Brown, author of *Play*, says that play is essential to our social skills, stress adaptability, intelligence, creativity, and problem-solving ability. Dr. Brown says that we can have "play" personality styles. There are the Collectors who like to collect things of interest; it can be social as in collectors of antique cars that take them to shows. Competitors are people who like to compete in either team sports or as lone competitors. The Creator/Artist could be a painter, a chef, or a songwriter. The Director might be an event planner, an exercise instructor, or a movie producer. The Explorer could be an astronaut, a ship captain, or a researcher trying to find a cure for cancer. The Joker could be a comedian, an entertainer, or class clown. Kinesthetics love to move, like dancers and athletes. Lastly, Storytellers might be a playwright, a screenplay writer, or a novelist.

Playing has many benefits besides reducing stress at any age. It can boost mental health and enhance cognitive function. It also helps promote creativity and innovation. Brené Brown says that as adults we struggle with resting and playing because of the stigma of *laziness*. Just like not needing much sleep is a "badge of honor" for some people, exhaustion and productivity in our culture is often a point of pride. We pride ourselves on our productivity and being busy, not realizing that this is a formula for disaster for our health. Remember the phrase, *"Pan metron ariston"*? Everything in moderation, including work. Work-life balance is an elusive goal that people are striving for these days. Remember to make time to play.

If you ever watched the *Friends* series in the nineties, there was an episode where Phoebe decided to run in Central Park like she ran when she was a kid with her arms and legs flailing about. Rachel was embarrassed to run with her because she looked weird, and Phoebe told her she didn't care what people thought because it made her feel free and it was fun! We need to give ourselves permission to feel free and to have fun.

Google started a trend in tech culture by making their office space more like a playground than a traditional stuffy office. Their organizational culture is designed to be an open environment that stimulates both collaboration and creativity. Many tech companies are following suit. They find that the type of environment that promotes play inspires innovation and creativity where employees are more engaged and purposeful. Promoting play is good for our brain because it ignites creativity.

As I discussed in Chapter 8, creativity is good for our brain and playing helps us be creative. Many themes in this book and foundations of health and wellness that I discuss overlap. Playing can overlap with breathing, moving, thinking, creating, and connecting.

If you have a hard time playing as an adult, here are some ideas.

1. Outdoor activities: combining breathing, creating, connecting with nature, and playing, i.e., geocaching, treasure hunts, hiking, ziplining, playing cornhole, flying kites, playing frisbee.
2. Creating and connecting with others, i.e., painting, crafts, collective storytelling, making plays, playing charades, dinner theater, karaoke, talent show, chalk art, building Legos with kids.
3. Movement and connecting with others, i.e., dance parties, dance classes, mini-golf, bowling, exercise classes, group fitness, yoga.
4. Thinking and connecting with others, i.e., game night, trivia, cards, checkers, mahjong, name that tune, escape room, murder mystery.

The list could go on and on. Use your imagination. The sky is the limit.

Key Points:

- Find ways to alleviate stress through play.
- Remember: when you stop playing, you start aging.
- Have fun and let go.
- Connect with friends and family and play together.
- Playing to destress is good for your health and well-being.

- Finding time to play is part of work life balance.
- Playing is needed at every age.

CHAPTER 13

Touch

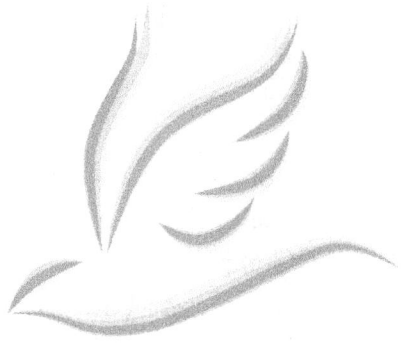

"*They will lay hands on the sick, and they will recover.*"
Mark 16:18

Why do babies stop crying when their parents pick them up and hold them? Why do we feel better when we are sad or sick once a loved one gives us a hug? Humans crave touch, which, as in Chapter 11, is really because we long for connection. Touch from another human is essential for our health and well-being. Even a kind touch from a stranger or a health professional can comfort us. I often touch my patients on the shoulder when I know they are feeling pain or discomfort. We often express our affection for one another with an embrace or hand holding. We greet one another with an embrace and say good-bye with an embrace.

I am a big fan of music, and everything reminds me of song lyrics (*in case you hadn't noticed*). Some lyrics that come to mind include "*Reach out and touch somebody's hand, make this world a better place if you can,*" by Diana Ross (1970). Not to mention a song by Neil Diamond that is known worldwide, yes, I'm talking about "Sweet Caroline." It's one of the most well-known sing-a-longs that I know of. Complete strangers will join hands at the sound of *"Hand, touching hand, reaching out, touching me, touching you."* Okay, I bet you are singing "Sweet Caroline" in your head right now.

Studies have shown that there is power in the human touch, yet it is one of our most underappreciated senses. Research suggests that oxytocin is released with physical touch. Oxytocin is known as "the love hormone" or the *bonding hormone*. Oxytocin reduces stress, fosters trust, and builds emotional connection. I believe that this is related to the power of God's love in us. Jesus put the expression of God's love into action when he healed people. In Luke 4:18, it says that Jesus came to heal the brokenhearted. Most of the healing that Jesus did was through touch. In Matthew 10:1, Jesus gave the power to heal sickness and disease to his followers. I believe we have the power to heal ourselves and to heal others within us. It might be belief, faith, or chemistry, but I'm living proof. When my liver failed, my aunt and uncle laid hands on me and prayed for my healing and I was healed.

I mentioned children in orphanages dying due to the lack of love and physical touch. I believe that humans don't walk immediately after birth like other species because of our need for physical touch. Babies are dependent on others for all of their needs, most of which involve touch by their parents or caretaker. This touch meets the need for love and security that is required for their healthy development. It's recommended that infants get skin to skin contact with their parents immediately after birth.

In Neonatal Intensive Care Units, they understand this well. Premature babies who require lifesaving surgery—like my oldest daughter, Jessica, who was born with gastroschisis (her intestines outside her body)—often spend months in the NICU. Jessica was there for five months. She had around the clock nurses who would hold her and the other babies as much as possible to fulfill their need for lifegiving and healing touch. This was forty years ago when they were much stricter about anyone being in the NICU besides nurses, so it was up to them to hold those babies. Parents were allowed in for very limited times, which was really difficult for me. Gastroschisis was a life-threatening defect that was not always repairable. It was a miracle and blessing that her repair went perfectly and was accomplished in one surgery.

Physical touch is not only healing and lifegiving, but it conveys empathy, warmth, and understanding. It also improves mental health because it can lower stress and anxiety. It is a universal language that transcends the spoken word. Touch builds and strengthens bonds in relationships. Consider massage therapy. Massage involves being touched by another person for therapeutic reasons. Through this touch, soft tissue is manipulated for the purpose of relaxation, promoting healing, relieving tension, stress and pain, improving circulation, draining lymphatics, and reducing inflammation.

Massage, even self-massage, should be a part of your self-care regimen. It can boost immunity and mental health. Lymphatic massage is a type of massage that helps detoxify the body. Breathing and bouncing (like on a trampoline or mini-rebounder) is a good way to stimulate the lymphatic system. Anything you can do to clear toxins from your body is beneficial to your health and well-being. Like most of the topics I cover, massage is beneficial for the body, mind, and spirit. It never ceases to amaze me that there are overlapping benefits for all the aspects of these foundational topics.

Michael Banissy, author of *Healing Touch*, reveals the research of why teams that high five each other win more games, why people who hug a lot are happier, and why a handshake makes it more likely you'll tell the truth to the person whose hand you are shaking. He writes about how we navigate life and the world around us with our sense of touch from in the womb and every minute we breathe. However, the sad fact is that there is a modern epidemic of "touch hunger" because people are more isolated than ever before, especially after the pandemic, where hugging became socially frowned upon.

Incidentally, for those of you with furry friends, studies also show that petting, touching, and holding animals releases oxytocin also. It has been shown to lower blood pressure and cortisol levels. Cortisol is a stress hormone. Remember what I said about chronic stress. Anything that can help manage stress is a good thing. Some hospitals and nursing homes as well as children's hospitals bring puppies in for patients and residents to hold. *Who doesn't feel happy holding a puppy?* There are many ways to improve mood and health that are practically free and easily accessible.

Key Points:

- Increase physical touch with loved ones, especially when you are feeling sick or down.
- Increase your faith in your innate power to heal.
- Add massage to your self-care regimen.
- Consider self-massage if you can't afford to go to a professional. Even putting lotion on and massaging it in is beneficial.
- Try dry brushing, breathing exercises, and rebounding to help stimulate your lymphatic system for detoxification.

CHAPTER 14

Hope

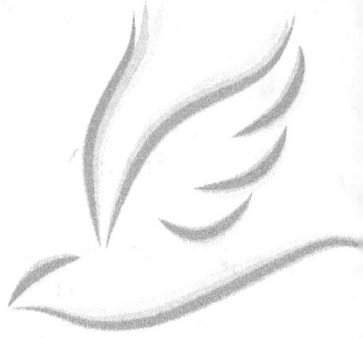

"Hope is being able to see that there is light despite all the darkness."
— Desmond Tutu

It saddens me to think that some young people today feel that the world and the future is too far gone, too hopeless, and too dark to bring children into. I don't agree. If we take a look at history, there have always been wars, famines, natural disasters, and dark times. In our somewhat recent history, there have been two world wars, the Great Depression, numerous floods, earthquakes, hurricanes, typhoons, influenza pandemics, and the list goes on.

In 1931, two million people were lost to the Yangtze River flood. Malaria has taken the lives of nearly five billion people. Smallpox and tuberculosis have each taken a billion lives. Today is no darker than any other time in history. In John 16:33, Jesus said, *"In this world you will have trouble, but take heart, I have overcome the world."* He is saying that no matter what is happening and how dark things seem, there is always hope. Hope springs eternal.

Hopelessness is a state of feeling powerless and helpless. Hopelessness can lead to mental, emotional, and physical illness. Fyodor Dostoevsky said, *"To live without hope is to cease to live."* To have hope is to be optimistic and have expectations of a favorable outcome. Hope is really about perspective. How a person perceives a situation tells a lot about who they are and how their future will be. As we discussed before, our minds are powerful and the reality that we believe is the reality we live. It's like a glass being half empty or half full. It's all about perspective.

The explorers that set out on an open ocean to find a new world had hope to keep pushing them on. Pioneers that crossed the plains and mountains to find a new and better life could have only done so with hope. When a young couple falls in love and starts a new life together, they have hope for a wonderful future together. Young athletes that aspire to go to the Olympics and win for their country can't practice for hours every day without hope.

Hope Rising, a book by Casey Gwinn, says that the science of hope can help us learn to overcome adversity, trauma, health crises, and life's struggles gleaned from over two thousand published studies. Life always finds a way. When it comes to our health, if we accept and buy into the false notion that we are going to eventually have whatever disease that others in our family had, we aren't operating in a hopeful mindset. The fact is our miraculous bodies have the power to heal if we believe they can and if we give them what they need to do so. There is Hope for Health, and just as I have laid out in this book, it isn't really that hard or complicated.

We simply have to recognize that nearly everything we need for a long healthy abundant life is free and available to us. It can be as simple as we make it. Breathe, Hydrate, Nourish, and Move for a healthy body. Think, Grow, Create, and Sleep for a healthy mind. Love, Connect, Play, Touch, and Hope for a healthy spirit. Life is a gift, and it should be cherished and not taken for granted. But like a forgiving parent who gives you grace when you mess up and fall short, our bodies are also forgiving. Don't feel like it's too late to change. It is never too late. There is always HOPE FOR HEALTH!

Key Points:

- You are not a victim of your biology.
- Optimism is free fuel for hope.
- Focus on the simple everyday things that can improve your health.
- Never lose hope.
- An attitude of gratitude can help feed our hopefulness.
- Hope changes your outlook in a positive direction.

Resources

Foundation

1. The American Academy of Oral Systemic Connection (AAOSH) https://www.aaosh.org
2. Chris Kammer, DDS, Founder of AAOSH. Minimally invasive, no drill dentist. Instagram @ drchrisk
3. Integrative Dental Medicine Scholar Society (IDMSS) https://www.idmscholarsociety.com
4. Dewitt Wilkerson DMS, Founder of IDMSS. Functional Dentist, Author of *The Shift: The dramatic movement toward health centered dentistry*. Educator, speaker wittwilkersondmd@gmail.com
5. American Dental Association (ADA) https://www.ada.org

Chapter 1 - Genesis?

1. Dale Bredesen, MD, Internationally recognized Neurologist. Chief science officer, Apollo Health. Author of *The End of Alzheimer's Program: The first protocol to enhance cognition and reverse cognitive decline*. @drdalebredesen

2. Richard Isaacson, MD, Internationally recognized Neurologist. Director of Alzheimer's Prevention Center. Author of *The Alzheimer's Prevention and Treatment Diet: Using nutrition to combat the effects of Alzheimer's Disease.*

3. VIOME. Health Intelligence Tests. https://www.viome.com Direct to consumer analytics.

4. Naveen Jain, Founder and CEO of VIOME. @naveenjainceo

5. Kiran Krishnan, Research Microbiologist. Co-founder and Chief Scientific Officer at Microbiome Labs. https://education.fxmed.co.nz/presenters/kiran-krishnan

6. Mike Czubiak, DDS, Speaker, President of AAOSH, author of *Hygiene Superstar*, https://www.hygienesuperstar.com/

7. Microbiome Labs https://www.microbiomelabs.com Gut microbiome testing, spore based probiotics and education.

8. Peter Attia, MD, Physician, Researcher of longevity medicine. Author of *Outlive: The Science & Art of Longevity.* @peterattiamd https://peterattiamd.com/

9. Ric Elias, CEO of Red Ventures and survivor of Flight 1549. @_ricelias

10. World Health Organization. https://www.who.int

Chapter 2 - Breathe

1. Atlas of the Mouth. Published by the American Dental Association in 1975 by Maury Massler

2. Bernard B. Baros, DDS, Practicing Dentist Widefield/Security Colorado, 32 years. July 24,1942- October 13, 2016

3. National Institute of Health (NIH) https://www.nih.gov

4. Louis Ignarro, PhD, Nobel Laureate, 1998. Discovery of nitric oxide as a signaling molecule. Author of *Dr. NO: The discovery that led to a Nobel prize and Viagra.*

5. Nathan Byan, PhD Biologist. https://www.drnathansbryan.com Author of *Functional Nitric Oxide Nutrition: Dietary strategies to prevent and treat chronic disease.*

6. Westin A. Price, DDS, Researcher and Author of *Nutrition and Physical Degeneration: A shocking and powerful testament to the adverse effects of modern processed diets upon health.*

7. Airway Health Solutions. https://www.airwayhealthsolutions.com Airway & Expansive Orthodontics Education.

8. The Breathe Institute. https://www.thebreatheinstitute.com Airway, sleep, breathing, health, growth, and development education.

9. The Vivos Institute. https://www.thevivosinstitute.com Comprehensive sleep and medicine mastery.

10. Patick McKeown, Breathwork Trainer and author of *Close Your Mouth*, *The Oxygen Advantage*, and *The Breathing Cure*.
11. Environmental Working Group (EWG). https://www.ewg.org Research and advocacy for removing toxins from our environment, agriculture, and water.
12. James Nestor, Investigative Journalist, Author of *Breathe: The new science of a lost art*. https://www.mrjamesnestor.com
13. Trish O'Herir, MS, RDH, International Speaker, Founder and President of O'Herir University and Author of *LipZip: Breath better to live better*. https://www.oheriruniversity.org
14. Wyndly: At home allergy testing and treatment direct to the consumer. https://www.wyndly.com
15. JonnyDiaz.Musicartist.Song:JustBreathehttps://www.youtube.com/watch?v=hnjeMwxFuBA

Chapter 3 - Hydrate

1. Dana Cohen, MD, Author of *Quench: Beat fatigue, drop weight, and heal your body through the new science of optimum hydration*. https://www.drdanacohen.com
2. C.W. Willington, MD, author of *Intracellular Hydration Breakthrough* and others.
3. Gina Bria, https://www.hydrationfoundation.org

Chapter 4 - Nourish

1. David Perlmutter, MD, author of *Drop Acid* and *Grain Brain: the surprising truth about wheat.* https://www.drperlmutter.com
2. Steven Gundry, MD, Author of *The Plant Paradox* https://www.drgundry.com
3. Robert Lustig, MD, Endocrinologist, and Author of *Metabolical, Fat Chance* and *The Hacking of the American Mind.* https://www.robertlustig.com He is also on the Advisory Board of Levels, a metabolic health platform.
4. Levels Health. https://www.levels.com A metabolic health platform leveraging the use of CGM's.
5. Casey Means, MD. Co-founder of Levels, health activists and Author of *Good Energy: The surprising connection between glucose metabolism and limitless health.* https://www.caseymeans.com
6. Senator Robert F. Kennedy Jr., environmental lawyer, politician & activist. @robertfkennedyjr
7. Mark Burhenne, DDS, Functional dentist, founder of FYGG and https://www.askthedentist.com https://www.fygg.com
8. Kami Hoss, DDS, founder of Super Mouth and author of *If Your Mouth Could Talk.* https://www.supermouth.com https://www.drkamihoss.com
9. Matt Callister, DMD, co-founder of Elementa Silver pH balancing products www.elementasilver.com. Discount Code: HOPE20

10. Simply Perio salivary test. https://www.https://simplytest.solutions/testing/saliva-perio-testing/ Administered by dental providers only.

11. Bristle Health salivary test. https://www.bristlehealth.com Direct to the consumer testing. Discount Code: HOPE10

12. Perio Protect Trays https://www.perioprotect.com Adjunctive periodontal therapy for home use. Available through dental professionals.

13. Power for Life: Superior Greenfood Plus http://www.terraoceana.com/shop/p/power-for-life

14. Emily Stein, PhD; Creator of Protektin by Primal Health LLC; https://www.dailydentalcares.com; Discount Code HOPE

15. *Need to Grow* documentary. https://www.grow.foodrevolution.org The need for regenerative agriculture.

16. Gabrielle Lyon, MD. Muscle centric physician, geriatric nutrition science and author of *Forever Strong: A new science-based strategy for aging well.* https://www.drgabriellelyon.com

17. William Li, MD, Author of *Eat to Beat Disease: The new science of how your body can heal.* https://www.drwillliamli.com

18. Jason Fung, MD, Nephrologist and Author of *The Complete Guide to Fasting: Heal your body through intermittent, alternate-day and extended fasting.* https://www.doctorjasonfung.com

Chapter 5 - Move

1. Peter Attia, MD, Physician, Researcher of longevity medicine. Author of *Outlive: The Science & Art of Longevity.* @peterattiamd
2. Emily Splichal, MD, Functional Podiatrist, Author of "Barefoot Strong: Unlock the Secrets of Movement Longevity" https://www.dremily-splichal.com/
3. Kelly McGonigal, PhD, Health Psychologist and Author of *Yoga for Pain Relief* and *The Joy of Movement.* https://www.kellymcgonigal.com

Chapter 6 - Think

1. Michelle Prince, Speaker, Publisher, and author of *Shine Through Your Story* and *Winning in Life Now.* https://www.michelleprince.com
2. Caroline Leaf, PhD, Neuroscientist, Speaker and Author of *Switching on Your Brain.* https://www.leaf.com

Chapter 7 - Grow

1. *Atomic Habits: An easy and proven way to build good habits and break bad ones* by James Clear https://www.jamesclear.com

Chapter 8 - Create

1. Scott Barry Kaufman and Carolyn Gregoire, Authors of *Wired to Create: Unraveling the mysteries of the creative mind.*
2. Jeff and Staney DeGraff, Authors of *The Creative Mindset: Mastering the six skills that empower innovation.*

Chapter 9 - Sleep

1. Sharon Moore, Speech Pathologist, Myofunctional Practitioner, and Author of *Sleep Wrecked Kids: Helping parents raise happy, healthy kids, one sleep at a time.* https://www.sleepwreckedkids.com
2. Mathew Walker, Neuroscientist and Author of *Why We Sleep: Unlocking the power of sleep and dreams.* https://www.sleepdiplomat.com

Chapter 10 - Love

1. Anna Machin, Evolutionary Anthropologist and Author of *Why We Love: The new science behind our closest relationships.* https://www.annamachin.com
2. Burt Bacharach, Hal David, songwriters. Composer and Lyricist of "What the World Needs Now Is Love Sweet Love." Sung by

Dionne Warwick. https://www.youtube.com/watch?v=FfHAs9cdTqg

3. Wei et al. Jul 2022. Greed personality traits lead to negative psychopathology and underlying neural substrates. *Social Cognitive and Affective Neuroscience.* https://doi.org/10.1093/scan/nsac046

Chapter 11 - Connect

1. Brené Brown, Researcher, Storyteller, Speaker and Author of *Atlas of the Heart: Mapping meaningful connection and the language of human experience, Imperfect: The gifts of imperfection,* and others. https://www.brenebrown.com

2. The Four Tops, music group. Song: "Reach Out and I'll Be There" written by Holland/Dozier/Holland and performed by The Four Tops - Reach Out (I'll Be There) (1967) HD 0815007

3. Kelly McGonigal, PhD, Health Psychologist, and Author of *The Science of Compassion: A modern approach for cultivating empathy, love and connection.*

4. Dan Buettner, Researcher, Explorer, Speaker, Author, and Producer of the Documentary *Live to 100: The secrets of the blue zones.* https://www.danbuettner.com

5. Joni Mitchell, Singer, Songwriter. Song: "Big Yellow Taxi." Joni Mitchell - Big Yellow Taxi (Official Lyric Video)

6. Earth Overshoot Day - https://www.footprint-network.org/our-work/earth-overshoot-day

7. J L Oshman, 2015. The effects of grounding (earthing) on inflammation, the immune response, wound healing, and prevention and treatment of chronic inflammatory and autoimmune diseases. *Journal of Inflammation Research.* Doi: https://doi.org/10.2147/JIR.S69656

8. *The Earthing Movie,* 2019 Documentary The Earthing Movie: The Remarkable Science of Grounding (full documentary)

9. Alexis Cowan, PhD, Molecular Biologist, Researcher @dralexisjazmyn

Chapter 12 - Play

1. Stuart Brown, MD. Author of *Play: How it shapes the brain, opens the imagination and invigorates the soul.* https://www.nifplay.org

2. Kelly McGonigal, PhD, Health Psychologist. Author of *The Upside of Stress: Why stress is good for you and how to get good at it.* https://www.kellymcgonagil.com

Chapter 13 - Touch

1. Diana Ross, Singer, 1970 Song: "Reach Out and Touch (Somebody's Hand)." Authors: Nikolas

Ashford and Valerie Simpson. Reach Out And Touch (Somebody's Hand)

2. Neil Diamond, Singer, Songwriter, 1969, "Sweet Caroline." Neil Diamond - Sweet Caroline (Audio)

3. Michael Banissy, Neuroscientist. Author of *Touch Matters: handshakes, hugs, and the new science how touch can enhance your well-being*.

Chapter 14 - Hope

1. Fyodor Dostoevsky, Russian Novelist, Essayist, and Journalist. Regarded as one of the greatest novelists in literature.

2. Casey Gwinn, J.D., President of Alliance for HOPE International, and Chan Hellman, PhD, Director of the Hope Research Center. Authors of *Hope Rising: How the science of hope can change your life*.

For anyone seeking a dental professional who shares many of the holistic, biological, and functional approaches, in this book, you can find recommendations at:

The International Academy of Biological and Dental Medicine (IABDM) I am certified through their Biological Hygienist program. Directory of Biological Providers: https://iaomt.org/search-by-region/

I am enrolled in the certificate program at the International Academy of Oral Medicine and Toxicology (IAOMT). https://iaomt.org/search-by-region/

For dental hygienists seeking Certification as an Oral Systemic Educator that can help promote medical dental integration:

The National Network of Healthcare Hygienists (NNHH) has an accredited Oral Systemic Educator (OSC) course to learn how to support your patients, with much of what I shared in this book. I am enrolled in this program. https://www.healthcarehygienists.org/blog/oral-systemic-educator-certificate-program

About the Author

I was fortunate enough to find a profession that is exactly what Vincent Van Gogh said a profession should be. He said, "Your profession is not what brings home your weekly paycheck, your profession is what you're put here on earth to do, with such passion and such intensity that it becomes spiritual in calling." Encouraging people to follow their dreams, find their purpose, improve their health and challenge themselves in all areas of their life is my passion. I dreamed of an idea that would bring *Hope for Health* to the world through understanding the oral systemic connection and whole body wellness. Starting a mobile hygiene practice to pursue that dream and share the message of *Hope for Health* with my patients was only the beginning. This book is another step in the pursuit of generating that *Hope for Health*.

I'd love to support you in any way I can. Here are ways to connect with me.

- 720-688-8028
- janet@hopeforhealthco.com
- https://www.hopeforhealthco.com
- https://www.instagram.com/hopeforhealthco/
- https://www.facebook.com/hopeforhealthco/#
- https://www.youtube.com/@hopeforhealthcolorado6032